You have lived many times

A journey in past lives

BRIGITTE CALLOWAY

DHP, Acc Hypnotherapist

A catalogue record for this book is available

from the National Library of New Zealand.

ISBN:
ISBN-13: 978-0-473-45965-9

To Miriam and Amos. You make my life beautiful!

CONTENTS

ACKNOWLEDGMENTS

Many may believe that a book is the creation of one person, the author, when in fact is the work of a team. I had many people in my team!

I would like to thank my husband Ian for the late evenings, sometimes nights, he spent reading my manuscript. By now, he may know it by heart. Without his encouragement, this book would have been just a lost project.

A huge thanks to my clients, who have entrusted me in guiding them through their past lives. What a journey! It was a privilege and honor to tell your stories!

I would also like to thank my clients who haven't been included in this book. Your time will come!

And, finally, my gratitude goes to my friend Charlotte for editing my manuscript.

.

Prologue

LIFE IS A MIRACLE

"There are only two ways to live your life: as though nothing is a miracle, or as though everything is a miracle."

Albert Einstein

I knew from a very early age that there must be something more to this life. I witnessed miracles that forced me to believe in the unbelievable. But never, in my wildest dreams did I believe I would witness others and myself traveling through past lives.

I grew up in Transylvania, the land of mysticism, in an Orthodox/ Greek Catholic family. Every Sunday morning my foster parents, who raised me from a very young age, dressed me in my Sunday best and took me to church. I am not very sure whether my dad had any connection with God, but my mom was a very religious woman. She wanted me to have a personal relationship with God. In our family, every celebration was about and around the church. Easters, Christmases, New Years, all the Saints' birthdays; according to the Greek Catholic calendar these were all reasons to be dragged to church. The Orthodox church had no Sunday school, so I had to sit on a cold bench in an old church with the elders, listening to something I didn't understand.

I was about 5 when I started being very curious about my mom's best friend, a lady who just lived next door. I noticed that every morning there was a queue in front of her gate, so I asked my mom why. She admitted, with embarrassment, that her friend was a fortuneteller. This intrigued me. I asked mom to tell me more, but this mysticism was antagonistic to her devout religious principles. However, in the years that followed, if any of us got sick or if there was a major problem in the family, our neighbor read cards for us. Very soon, I had the privilege of seeing her in action. In hindsight, I now realize that I've never come across such an accurate Tarot reader. She predicted names, dates and events with precision. This lady, my mom's best friend, was a nun in a monastery in the former Czechoslovakia and learnt Tarot from one of the older sister wives of Christ. In the late 1950s, her order was dissolved because most of the nuns were believed to have stepped on the Devil's path; some read Tarot, others talked to spirits or saw ghosts. To avoid forming a cult, the church dispersed the nuns over Eastern Europe. Mom's friend was sent to Transylvania. As a child, this very gifted lady told me stories about life after life, spirits and angels. I was like a sponge absorbing all the information I could. I had already figured out that this was to be my path, my career and my destiny….

In my early 20s, I bought an old Volkswagen. I was so proud of my first car. However, bad luck followed me. Frequently, outings in my new Volkswagen involved accidents, none attributed to my driving ability rather to that of other road users. I was even hit by cars when parked on the side of the road. Every accident was quite serious and I thought there must be something wrong with the car or with me. I heard about an old man living in a small village in the mountains, who cleared cars of bad spirits. At least that's what I was told. So, one Sunday, I drove to meet him… fortunately without incident. Many others sought out this car whisperer. It seemed I was not alone in owning a cursed vehicle. He lived in a very poor village. He greeted those wishing for blessing whispering something to each in turn. When he got to me, he told me that I would never have another accident. And I didn't. He also told me that my destiny was to see beyond what is. I wondered for a while what he meant. Now I know!

In that same year I witnessed a yogi levitating. I became involved in a meditation movement, which was quite odd for the society I was part of. Not only odd, but also illegal! The group was led by some Russian yogis, who spent time in my town. The yoga they taught was far removed from that accepted in Western society. In their last days with us, these Russians talked about the power of the mind and how they, and us too, could control everything if we put our minds to it. That's when I witnessed them levitating. By then, I stopped wondering and accepted that everything, or rather nothing, was as it seemed. I now believe in miracles and I now know that there is so much more to this life than our recognized five senses can grasp.

In my mid 20s, I met a girl, just a few years younger than me, who claimed to be a clairvoyant. I was very intrigued, as the girl appeared to be unexceptional. There was nothing paranormal about her! So, one evening, I visited her and she agreed to 'channel'. I remember that there was a candle on her table and, as she tuned in, the flame started to dance. Shapes of faces and bodies started to manifest in the flame. That's when I saw the distinct image of my auntie who had just passed away. Her face in that flame was so clear. She even started moving her mouth as if she wanted to tell me something. The girl channeled the messages and everything seemed so normal. Just the way it should have been!

For many years I endeavored to learn more about what seemed intangible, yet so real, but just beyond my field of vision, about divine and creation. I went to church, I meditated, I read about New Age, which wasn't an established practice in my country, I read the bible and other divination books belonging to all sorts of religions and I spent years studying philosophy at university. None gave me an accurate answer, so, at some stage in my life, I decided to put them all behind me and start fresh… with an urge to discover what exactly was outside of my inner life and how I could get to that level of consciousness to positively affect the collective consciousness.

In New Zealand, I started working in Hypnotherapy, being involved at the beginning with medical cures. I helped people who wanted to quit smoking or wanted to lose weight, and others suffering from depression, anxiety, chronic pains, migraines and phobias. You name it. I've done them all. Around that time, I came across some past life regression books and I became fascinated and intrigued. By then, I was teaching workshops in chakra balancing, the law of Attraction, karma, mindfulness and meditation. I was, in fact, deeply spiritual, in the search of developing my own consciousness and putting my fingerprint on others. Therefore, I began studying past life regression and since then I have never looked back.

Client after client proved to me that there were many other shapes, forms and stages of the soul's existence. With every session, I got more deeply involved in researching and proving this point. I too have regressed into past lives and the experiences were so real whilst past life memories so vivid. Man or woman, young or old, in Europe, America, Asia or Africa, my soul recognized the one I was.

This book is about the memories of my clients, in one-on-one or group past life regressions, as well as my own experiences in this field. For me, there is no doubt that our eternal souls have travelled in time and that we have all lived many times. All the cases presented in this book have been recorded during past life regressions sessions under hypnosis.

For privacy reasons, some of the names have been

changed. In the hypnotic dialogue with my clients, I will refer to myself as using the initials of my name BC.

THE SOUL'S EVOLUTION

"My life often seemed to me like a story that has no beginning and no end"

Carl Jung

Many people are afraid of hypnosis. They believe that, perhaps whilst under, the therapist can make them walk like a drunk chicken or say weird things. That's not the case though. Hypnotherapy is in fact a state of deep relaxation and of focused consciousness. If you have ever meditated, you would know exactly what I mean. What is important to know is that, whilst under hypnosis, you are still aware and in control.

To induce a hypnotic state, a creative therapist uses all sorts of induction and trance deepening techniques. People react differently to them. Some are better subjects and more susceptible to hypnosis, others more skeptical and resist longer. At the end of the day, I have no doubt that everybody can be hypnotized. You may disagree, but I can prove the fact that you have already experienced hypnosis at some stage in your life. Have you ever driven your car on a beautiful sunny day, in such a state of relaxation and peace that, when arriving to the destination, you couldn't remember how you got there? You may have thought that the music on the radio took your focus away, but in fact you experienced what we call *"highway hypnosis"*.

This book is not a manual for hypnotherapists, thus my intention is not to go into details about methods of inducing hypnosis. However, what I really want to pass on to all my readers is that a journey to past lives is not possible if the client doesn't achieve deep hypnosis.

At the beginning of my career as a hypnotherapist, I used scripts that were written by more experienced therapists than I. In time, I learnt that there was no right or wrong method as long as I could induce hypnosis. Therefore, I wrote my own scripts and later I learnt to improvise according to each client.

You may ask yourself if one can recall memories from past lives in the absence of hypnosis. Well, my answer is no because, for you to be able to remember, your brain activity has to be based on theta waves. You see, there are four different brain waves that measure the electrical activity of our brains: alpha, beta, theta and delta. Us humans function in beta activity, a state of complete awareness and we kick to alpha when we are relaxed or close our eyes. Do you remember the highway hypnosis? This is always a state of daydreaming in alpha activity. Delta brain activity is related to sleeping, when we tap into the unconsciousness. Theta brain waves are what we – hypnotherapists – work with. It is also our brain activity when we meditate. In both hypnosis and meditation, the subconscious part of our brains dominates.

So, a regression into past lives starts with hypnosis. Once the client is under hypnosis, I start their journey to a significant past life, one that is unconsciously chosen by the client and one that makes sense to them. It is also a lifetime that was made possible by a specific issue carried on in the present life. I record every session and there is always something new to discover when reviewing the tapes.

For me, the regression itself is the proof that we have lived many lives as women or men of different races, nationalities and skin colors. In each life, we earn our existence working in different fields and belonging to various hierarchies, religions and traditions. We may have been married or single, rich or poor, healthy, sick or handicapped. We may have lived and died in cultures we or perhaps no one has ever heard of before. We may have died of natural causes, young or old, or we may have had traumatic deaths. We've been through all sorts of scenarios.

Our soul is eternal, whilst our spirit, that makes our being, is individual. We may have been through all the possible combinations of humanity and, if we haven't already, we will still return until we have learnt all the lessons our soul is supposed to experience. I don't believe that these lessons are randomly chosen. I rather believe that our soul chooses the lesson it desires to learn in the next life together with the family within which it wishes to incarnate. Therefore, the soul identifies the circumstances where a particular lesson is more than likely to be learnt. To be more specific, our soul decides first of all if it wants to come back. It is all about choice and evolution.

With every life and every lesson learnt, the soul evolves. Is it possible to learn everything and be totally pure and complete? To be honest, I cannot answer this question because I have never regressed a person to a life of perfection. However, I cannot deny the fact that there are master souls that may have reached excellence perhaps by being able to learn every possible lesson faster. They may have been chosen at the world's conception or they may just have been avid learners.

The way I have witnessed that this evolution takes place is by starting in the space between two lives, referred to as "life between lives", a place where souls feel at home. This is a special place where souls have a great connection to the higher energy, referred to as *"all that it is"*, or to heal after a life lived on earth. It is also a realm where souls determine their next incarnation.

It is in this energetic level where the soul picks the family and the lesson to be learnt in the next life. Any of the karmic lessons, spirituality, independence, trust, love and so many more, could represent journeys to explore in the next incarnation. I have spent years studying karmic lessons and I conclude that each of them has a multitude of facets. Just think of independence/ freedom being a lesson for our souls. Freedom comes in many ways. It can be a personal freedom, a professional one or even a creative or artistic freedom. It also can be a freedom of mind or of a physical nature. Freedom relates to breaking all the chains that may constrict us or may narrow our existence. A soul may need several lives to go through all the aspects of freedom. Also how many facets has love; or balance or even temptation or addiction? Therefore it is the soul's duty and desire to learn little bits of a lesson until it is fully understood and completed. At the end of the day, the soul evolves in the aim of perfection.

Without claiming that I fully understand the complexity and the make up of our souls, my conclusion is that karma as well as the law of Attraction are tools the soul can use in order to travel from one existence to another and to evolve. Again, without declaring that I hold the answer to why souls decide over one lesson and not another, one thing is clear to me: souls are in charge of choosing a family, a group and, why not, even a destiny.

It is said that souls reincarnate in the same groups, which is partially true. The soul groups are necessary for souls to feel familiarity in a lifetime. This is where déjà vu comes in. People involved in our lives today may have well been part of our past existences. We may have played different roles in each other's lives and crossed paths in other existences in order to help each other learn, teach and evolve.

Many of my clients have recalled people in past lives who play important roles in their present life. They have mentioned that these people may have looked totally different, but they were still able to recognize their energy.

This happens only because souls recognize other souls.

HOW WE REMEMBER

*"Everything becomes and recurs eternally; escape is
impossible"*

Nietzsche

To understand how we recall memories, we first need to
know how our brains work. For the purpose of hypnosis
only, I would say that our brains have two parts, the
conscious mind and the subconscious mind. We often
believe that our conscious part is the strongest part of our
brain, in charge of all that is, but in fact this is not true. Our
conscious mind is the weakest part of our brain. We spend
almost the whole day in this part, therefore we think,
analyze and rationalize with the weakest part of our brain.

The conscious mind includes a rational component

17

which is not always correct, a willpower part which is temporary, an analytical part which tries continuously to figure how to sort things out, and a temporary memory which is in fact very limited. The conscious mind can only hold a limited amount of memory or data at one time. To be more specific, not more than seven chunks of data. So, we rely day by day on this very frail part of the brain.

On the other hand, the subconscious is powerful. The subconscious mind is home to the Autonomic Nervous System, the permanent memory, imagination, feelings, emotions, beliefs, and habits. They all help us achieve goals and aim for success. And because it is so powerful, the subconscious stores all our memories for an unlimited amount of time, starting with our first day of life. All the memories are stored in the subconscious in the same way data is stored on a computer hard drive, thus if you know how a hard drive stocks up data, you know exactly what I mean!

The way we access memories is incredible. Just imagine yourself listening to the radio and noticing that most of the songs are triggers for some memories. A song may bring back the first kiss or perhaps the day you were dumped by a lover, or an exam or your wedding day. Every song you know is an anchor for a feeling and the memory that relates to it. Remember though that the memory you recall may be distorted or generalized because of the filters used in accessing it. These filters are the memories themselves, your own value and beliefs system, your decisions and the Meta Programs. These programs are our own representations of every experience.

As people's perception of life is different, the way they relate to information is also different. It is common for two people to remember the same memory from a totally different perspective, based on their own representational systems. For some people a memory is triggered by an image or sound, for others by a smell, taste or even a feeling. Also, the same memory can trigger different feelings in two individuals.

As I've said, for the purposes of hypnosis only, we refer to two parts of the human mind: the conscious and the subconscious. However, Sigmund Freud, the founder of psychoanalysis, divided the brain into three levels: conscious, subconscious, which he called pre-conscious, and unconscious. According to Freud, the conscious mind occupies 10% and works as a scanner of information; the subconscious 50 – 60% and stores every recent memory and the unconscious mind 30 – 40% and stores every past or long-term memory. In the same way, Freud argued that the human psyche or personality has three main aspects, id, ego and superego, all developing at different stages of our existence. Freud's theory about the human mind has never been validated, at least not scientifically, but, to be perfectly honest, it would be very difficult to be proven by science. As much as this was criticized or acclaimed, I personally take from it the fact that there is a very organized way the human brain stores information and the certainty that the same mind has the ability to remember every memory created by an experience.

I believe that we can remember everything. We have the right brain structure, the capacity of the subconscious mind to store huge amounts of information for an unlimited time and we have a cell memory. Would that mean that we store information at the cellular level? More than likely! Just remember the saying *"it's like riding a bike"*. I am sure you have heard this many times. Once you have learnt to ride a bike, you never forget it. You may have also heard about *"muscle memory"* which refers to the fact that a muscle would remember how to do a certain activity even if you hadn't performed it for a long time. You don't have to learn to walk again after a prolonged period of incapacitation, for example a broken leg healing in a cast for a long period of time. Once the cast is removed, one may walk with caution, but the walking ability is stored as data in your brain. Your leg muscles would also remember that they walked prior to the injury and they would access the memory naturally.

I have no doubt that the human brain can remember everything, from the womb up until the present. I have regressed clients to their childhood time, to memories that seemed forgotten or hidden. I have also regressed clients to the time spent in their mother's womb.

Are we really able to remember memories from past lives too? We sure are. Our past lives' memories are stored at our eternal soul level. Your soul holds all your memories from every past life you have lived.

HIDDEN MEMORIES

"Memory is the mother of all wisdom"

Aeschylus

Our brains are very similar to a computer hard drive. Every experience that makes up a memory is stored for a later use exactly as a computer stores every saved document for the time when we need to access it. In the sensory stage, which lasts for a fraction of a second, a memory is created and then stored as a short-term memory, and after filtered, stored as a long-term memory. For a memory to be transformed to a long-term memory, it needs to be used or utilized and repeated. The more we know about a subject, the easier it becomes to connect a new memory to already stored information.

Just imagine yourself in front of your computer. It is more than likely to save a photo of a mountain in an already existing folder called "landscape" rather than in one called "cars" because of associating the photo with others saved in a certain folder. Therefore, one of the most important aspects in recalling or retrieving a memory is association.

In the same way, the context that a certain event took place can help recalling a specific memory as well as the feelings or emotions one had whilst experiencing the event that created a memory. There is an important aspect that involves the feelings one had in regards to an experience. This is based on the fact that we cannot store at the same time two opposite memories, one positive and one negative for instance, about the same experience. It has to be either positive or negative, depending on which is stronger, but never the two together. In the same way, we cannot store simultaneously two antagonistic memories about an event that triggered two opposite feelings.

I am sure that you are already asking yourself why some memories are hidden from us, if the brain works so wonderfully and perfectly in storing each memory. Just think about the trauma that some of our stored memories may cause once they are triggered or accessed. Our brains make sure that we don't live permanently in a panic or an anxiety mode. You may also argue that anxiety is an epidemic these days and that there are many people suffering from panic attacks. Therefore let me clarify that anxiety disorder is just a normal response to stress in general or extremely stressful situations, and that panic attacks are part of the same anxiety spectrum and are triggered by specific external factors. However, none of them mean living constantly in anxiety or panic mode.

Hypnotherapy helps retrieve hidden memories in a therapy called regression. Whether it is an earlier moment in the present life or even in a past life, these memories can easily be accessed and reframed or reformatted if it is required. Imagine again the way your files are stored on your computer. The extension of a file can always be reformatted or changed according to where you want to use it and how much free space the hard drive has.

There is no difference really between a regression to an earlier time in the present life and a past life regression, except the period of time regressed to. Both processes are regressions to memories that could well be forgotten or hidden. All memories that don't appear to be readily accessible may possibly be traumatic, painful or just not important for today's context. In all these cases, opposition to recalling a memory is very strong. I will give you as an example my husband's regression to his childhood.

My husband Ian is an artist and spent all his life painting. You may say that, being involved in visual arts, the representational system he relies on to express himself is definitely visual. But you're wrong. His whole perspective is more emotional, which makes him a kinesthetic person. Anyway, my husband had a very weird condition that affected his ability to do what he did best, painting. For the last few years, very often he had odd breathing problems that couldn't be attributed to any recognized medical respiratory conditions.

Being regressed to an earlier time in his childhood, all that he could see was *"a green field and a tree in the middle of the field"*. He was able to feel the energy of himself, running on the grass and looking at the field. However, he wasn't the one visualizing himself running; he recalled this memory as looking through somebody else's eyes. He knew that that person was a child of a similar age, but he couldn't recognize him.

In the second regression, Ian saw the same scenery, but this time he remembered himself, at the age of 11, climbing the tree. Again, the memory was recalled through the unknown child's eyes. This time though, Ian remembered falling from the tree.

It was at the third session when Ian associated this fall and the sinus and respiratory condition he has more recently suffered from. Ian recalled the incident, remembering how he fell three or so meters onto his back and injured himself severely, whilst having the same shortness of breathing that he has in the present. This perhaps may be contributing to the symptoms of his yet undiagnosed condition. The point is not whether his condition was or was not caused by an emotional and physical incident when he was 11. The point is that in hypnosis, every suggestion creates less opposition. In Ian's case, opposition to the painful memories, by visualizing them through another person's eyes and recalling just fragments of them, got weaker with each session. Therefore, remembering bits of a memory, or totally opposing to recall it, doesn't mean that the memory is not stored.

The same phenomenon relates to past life regressions. Once a memory is identified, it can be recalled. The reason why we cannot naturally access memories from past lives is based on the fact that we cannot necessarily associate them with memories from the present life: memories which are less cognitive, have less context or association are less likely to be remembered without a stimulus. It is just the normal way our brain works. However, the whole regression process creates the necessary trigger to bring the memory back.

PHYSICAL PAIN FROM A PAST LIFE

"I am certain that I have been here as I am now a thousand times before, and I hope to return a thousand times."

Goethe

I met Simon a few months ago at one of the open-minded people groups in my area. Run once a month by different people, the group was a meeting place for spiritual individuals. The rule was that the organizer decided on the topic and, for two hours, people just chatted around the subject. Simon was an energy healer and the discussions were about different energy healing techniques. I was so happy to attend because I was new to the city and I didn't know too many people. My husband and I had just moved a few weeks ago from a little town five hours away. I was also recovering from surgery on my ankle, so any distraction was gratefully received.

Very calm, funny, with big blue eyes, Simon was just a big soft bear. During the meeting, we got quite friendly and later that evening, when my husband and I were about to leave, I gave him my business card. A few days later, he rang and booked an appointment. Just like that!

He arrived on a Monday just after lunch and he brought his partner with him. I don't mind additional people attending if my clients feel they need support. Simon filled in the forms and said that he was curious about his past reincarnations. On the other hand, for the last ten years, he had a weird lower back pain that refused to go away. He believed that the cause of it might have been in one of his past existences. He also said that he had seen doctors, specialists, healers but nothing took his pain away. Listening to Simon, I realized that he suffered from a phantom pain, which is a discomfort or pain with no medical reasons.

He was the easiest subject to hypnotize so I proceeded rapidly through the induction stage and deepening the state of trance. I asked him to imagine himself traveling on an escalator that went many levels down. In just a few minutes, Simon started answering my questions.

"I wear army boots. Old army boots... old and shiny.... My palms are so dirty. I am young, just 21. My palms are so dirty...", he said and then he started speaking very fast. Words just came out of his mouth one after another.

Simon: *"Phillip. My name is Phillip. I have a father who is still alive, yep, he is. Big family, many siblings, but I have no girlfriend."*

Suddenly he started being anxious, so I tried distracting him.

BC: *"Now I want you to look around and notice the surroundings. What do you see; where are you?*

Simon: *"I don't know. It's dark and foggy. It's a scary silence. I hear the silence. It's scary. I am fighting. I am very nervous.... We are all nervous. There are people behind me... all nervous..."*

I knew he was scared. His face showed it and his voice grew deeper and deeper. He almost whispered.

BC: *"That's OK. Nothing can touch you. Just float above the scene if that makes you feel more comfortable."*

Simon: *"It's 1940. I don't speak English. I speak French... Yes, I am in France. I enrolled in the war. We were all doing it.... for our country...."*

BC: *"Are there any people around you?"*

Simon: *"There is so much death around me... death everywhere. I am scared, really scared... I am alone where I am."*

BC: *"That's fine. Now, as I count down from five to one, I want you to go to a relevant scene in that lifetime. 5 going further to a scene you can choose, 4, 3 just remembering whatever comes to your mind, 2 and 1. As you are finding yourself in a significant scene in that lifetime, I want you to look around. Where are you?"*

Simon: *"In a bunker... hiding... people killing people.... I am reading a letter. I don't know where from, but I see the letter in my hands. Others are reading too. We all have letters from our dear ones."*

BC: *"What else do you see?"*

Simon: *"There are many men around me. Some are still alive. No point making friends! We are here for a short time."*

Simon got stuck in that moment. He started being more anxious and I had the feeling that he couldn't move forward in time. I decided that this was the right time to take him to the moment when death occurred, so I guided him to the very last moments of his lifetime as Phillip.

Simon: *"I am walking across a field. The sun is*

coming up. It should be around 6am. There are explosions. There are bodies flying in the air. Bang! The explosion hit the ground. I fly in the air."

His face became calm, relaxed and I even noticed a smile on his lips. Simon enjoyed the release of his soul.

BC: *"That's fine. You are safe and nothing can touch you. What do you see, feel or sense now?"*

Simon: *"It's so nice, so much peace. There are angels around me; very nice. The silence has a sound to it. Very weird... I hear the music, but I know that there is none."*

BC: *"What else is happening?"*

Simon: *"Angels talking to me. Yep, they are. They say: just breathe... You are always loved...."*

BC: *"Do they say anything about the lesson you decided to learn in that lifetime? Or perhaps you can recall that particular lesson."*

Simon: *"I can do it. I don't have to be afraid. I can do it! We can do everything we want to do!"*

BC: *"Anything else?"*

Suddenly, Simon's face changed color and he got even more relaxed. A few minutes later, his closed eyes started moving rapidly and I already knew that he jumped straight into another life.

Simon: *"I see buildings now. Feels like London. 1814 is the year. It's so busy..."*

BC: *"Feels like London?"*

Simon: *"I see it clearly now. It is London. I recognize every building"*

Simon has never been to London. Actually he has never traveled outside of New Zealand. However, he recognized a city he has never seen in his present life.

BC: *"As you are now looking down to your feet, what do you wear?"*

Simon: *"Nice pair of shoes. I am old. I am in my eighties. I am a man.... rich man with a big family. My wife has passed. Childbirth... That makes me feel sad."*

BC: *"You have a family and friends perhaps. Is there anybody you recognize?"*

Simon: *"Yep. Leah is there. She is my little girl... not so little anymore. She is in her late 30s. She is courting somebody. She has curly hair."*

When she heard her name, Leah started crying.... and smiling. Leah is Simon's partner in the present life. They met later in life when their marriages fell apart. They have two children each.

BC: *"Is it a happy lifetime?"*

Simon: *"Very. I worked with ships and I made good*

money. I am really settled. Life wasn't a struggle. I have a nice family and I am happy; unfortunately my wife died giving birth... long time ago."

I decided to move Simon backwards in time, perhaps to a time when he was younger.

Simon: *"I am holding a baby. My son. I don't remember his name but I know my name. Thomas. He is beautiful. My wife is still alive. Her name is Samantha. I love her with all my heart. I work hard for the family. What a beautiful life!"*

BC: *"Do you recognize your son? Is he somebody you know in your present lifetime?*

Simon: *"Yep. He is Alice, my friend from now. He looks different, but I know he is Alice."*

BC: *"Now, as I count back from five to one, I want you to find yourself in the very last day of that life, without any stress, without judging or hurting, just noticing the event. 5, 4, 3, 2, 1.... Find yourself in the last few moments in that existence as Thomas. Where are you?"*

Simon: *"I am in bed. I am not sick, but I know that my time is now. Kids are around me. Leah is there.... but not there.... Her kids are. I am very, very old. I just die now of old age...now."*

Simon's face changed again. He was at peace. I

could tell that his soul left his body.

BC: *"That's fine. Rest and float above the scene and whenever you're ready, tell me what you see."*

Simon: *"Everything is light. There are angels around me. They tell me go to my mom. I don't know what they mean. Wait. I know.... they tell me that I am home again! They say I have done everything right. There are masters too. Many people are there.... not people, just entities. The masters are not saying anything to me. Just looking down at me. They are happy, overjoyed with how I lived. They are writing things about my life in a book. They are very happy."*

BC: *"Is there any lesson you learnt? Is there anything you want to share with me?"*

Simon's voice changed suddenly. He became prophetic.

Simon: *"Love, just love. You can succeed if you figure love out."*

I have seen Simon many times since the regression. I have also followed his work and evolution. I don't remember though hearing him complain about the back pain that harassed him for more than ten years. Would this be because he healed himself by going back in time, into a lifetime where an injury may have occurred, as Simon recalled breaking his spine in the last moments as Phillip? I don't hold the key, but I am sure that Simon's soul knows the answer.

REINCARNATION AND KARMA

"I am confident that there truly is such a thing as living
again, that the living spring from the dead, and that the
souls of the dead are in existence"

Socrates

If you believe that your soul is eternal and immortal, then you already believe in reincarnation. This concept may be a relatively new idea in Western society, but it has been around for many centuries in other parts of the world. Hinduism, for instance, bases its concept on reincarnation.

The Vedic hymns, which are the oldest collection of Hindu texts, indicate that after death, the soul returns home to a heavenly existence or afterlife and, after a while, experiences another death. The Upanishads, which are philosophical texts included in the Vedas, in the 9th Century BC, came up with the concept of the soul returning to live again after the second death. This second incarnation of the soul is actually based on karma and Samsara. I am sure that you have all heard of karma, the law of cause/effect. Samsara, on the other hand, relates to being born all over again, or in other words, continuously passing from a life to another one.

For Buddhism, the soul is not necessarily eternal; each time it reincarnates, a new individuality is formed and the knowledge acquired in previous lives is passed on. Therefore the knowledge accumulates life after life. However, this new entity does not hold on to the lessons already learnt in previous existences. Therefore, enlightenment is not permanent for Buddhism. Just imagine it like this: a new person evolves from a previous one, both different, but both identical at the same time. When you look carefully into it, the concept is crystal clear. Just picture a mother and her daughter or perhaps twin siblings. They are different, but according to their bloodline, they are alike. For adepts of Buddhism, karma for kindness or punishment carries on.

Reincarnation and karma are concepts denied by Christianity and other religions too. For Christians, there is only one life, the one we live at the present and the one that ends once death occurs, followed by a heavenly eternal afterlife. For Christianity, a place in heaven or hell is secured based on the choices made in this life. For me though this is just another way of perceiving the law of cause/effect.

The concept of karma is strongly related to reincarnation. This is perhaps the reason why many of my clients booked past life regression sessions. There was a curiosity about their karma accumulated in other lives. Some believed that they may have acted against ethical values in one or more past lives and karma bites them in the present. The truth is that karma is not a law of punishment. It is just an effect of a certain cause. Perhaps the best statement regarding karma is Newton's law of cause/ effect: " *For every action there is an equal and opposite reaction* ".

Most people refer to good and bad karma. According to them, positive attracts good and negative attracts bad. I believe that *"likes attract likes"* is an indication of the presence of the Law of Attraction rather than karma.

At the end of the day, who are we to judge what is good and what is bad. These concepts are relative. I always give my clients the example of a German man who, in World War II, hid a family of Jewish people. When the authorities knocked on his door and asked if there were any Jews in his house, he answered no. He saved the lives of the Jewish family. Did that bring a flow of good karma? Perhaps, but what about the lie he said? Did that generate bad karma? Where can we draw the line between good and bad?

Karma and the Law of Attraction are different concepts. Karma refers to action, whilst the Law of Attraction mostly to thoughts. You can picture karma as being active or physical and the Law of Attraction being mental or emotional. The two work together up to a point.

Many of my clients want to be regressed in the hope of identifying and even changing karma accumulated in past lives. Most of them don't know that there is no way of stopping karma that is already in action. Experiencing this karma, called Prarabdha, is inevitable because it is already set in motion. No matter how hard you try, you cannot stop this avalanche once it has already started.

We refer to the sum of karma accumulated in every life we already lived as Sanchita. This is formed by many so-called Agami karmas, one for each life. Agami is the karma accumulated in the current life, but remember that we have lived many lives that were current at some stage. Therefore, we cannot change Prarabdha, because, as I have said, it is already ruling our life; however we can change Agami, the karma we are accumulating at the moment and therefore influence Sanchita. At the end of the day, we should act always for a positive outcome, without even focusing on karma in general.

Whether you believe in reincarnation or not is up to you. For me though, reincarnation is proven. I don't sympathize with any religions, but I am a spiritual being, who knows that there must be more to life than this reality. I admire and respect people who have a strong belief based on their religion. I am not one of them though. I am open to possibilities!

THE TRUTH ABOUT CURSES

"Doctrine of reincarnation is neither absurd nor useless. It is not more surprising to be born twice than once"

Voltaire

Diane called me on a Saturday early in the morning. Normally, at that time, I would have been sleeping. But I wasn't. I had to teach a workshop on the Law of Attraction that morning, so I was preparing my lecture.

When the phone rang, I thought to myself that this could be somebody very keen, maybe desperate, to call and book an appointment so early on a Saturday. I was right. Diane introduced herself and started talking about her suspicion in regards to a kind of curse, perhaps relating to bad karma or maybe a blockage she carries from a past incarnation. Very shy and respectful, she said that there was a story in her family about a curse that haunted many ancestors. She mentioned a few times a possible curse, thus I knew that she really believed in it. We booked the appointment and a few days later, Diane came to my practice to be regressed.

She was a beautiful young girl and I realized how right I was about her. Diane was shy and very polite. She seemed very concerned in regards to her future...as we all do, to be perfectly honest. Like many young people, despite her talents and knowledge, Diane couldn't decide what her next step was going to be. She told me that she wanted to study, but couldn't put her finger on a subject she really liked. She had desires and dreams, but she seemed blocked by external forces. Just a very beautiful, nice person concerned about life in general!

Diane was the ideal client to hypnotize, so she reached a trance state very quickly.

BC: *"What do you see, feel or hear?"*

Diane: *"It's dark. Very dark."*

BC: *"Can you see yourself? Is there anything you can see in the dark?"*

Diane: *"Nothing. It's dark. But I hear a noise."*

BC: *"What noise is that?"*

Diane: *"Like someone stumbling."*

BC: *"Are there people around you?"*

Diane: *"No. I'm alone. I don't see anybody. It's just me..."*

BC: *"How does that make you feel?"*

Diane: *"I am very scared. It's so dark..."*

BC: *"There's nothing to be scared about. What do you see or feel around you?"*

Diane: *"I am a woman and I am 30 years old. My name is Amy. I think that I am in a shed. It is very damp and dark. It is somewhere outside. I also know that my dress is beige."*

BC: *"Do you have a boyfriend or a husband as Amy?"*

Diane: *"I have a husband, but I don't remember his name. I don't like him at all."*

BC: *"Why is that?"*

Diane: *"He locked me in the shed. He is not happy. I have done something and he is not happy about it."*

BC: *"What have you done?"*

Diane: *"I lost something.... I lost my baby."*

BC: *"How did that happen?"*

Diane: *"My baby girl died at birth. It's not my fault, but he keeps me locked in the shed. He believes that the baby died because of me. It's not my fault though."*

BC: *"Do you know what year it is?"*

Diane: *"It should be 1919. I am somewhere in Europe and I speak a different language."*

BC: *"Do you love your husband?"*

Diane: *"No, I don't. He is a bad man. I married him because I was told to. I want to leave him, but I cannot. I am locked in the shed."*

BC: *"That's fine. Don't worry too much."*

Then, I started counting down and slowly moved her to another scene in that lifetime.

BC: *"What do you see, feel or hear?"*

Diane: *"I left my husband. I am now 42. I live in another house. It's definitely not the same house."*

BC: *"Whose house is it?"*

Diane: *"It's my friend Luke's. He is an old friend. I've known him for years."*

Luke was Diane's friend in the present life.

BC: *"What do you do there?"*

Diane: *"I clean. I am upset as I kept running from my husband."*

BC: *" Look at yourself and describe what you see."*

Diane: *"I have long brown hair and blue eyes. Very long hair…"*

BC: *"Do you have a new boyfriend or husband?"*

Diane: *"No boyfriend. I don't want another husband!"*

BC: *"What about children?"*

Diane: *"No, my baby girl died. I named her Alice. I am sad that she died!"*

BC:*" Don't be. It's all fine."*

I instructed Diane to move forward even further in time and to visit her last day as Amy.

BC: *"Where are you now?"*

Diane: *"I am outside. I am old, maybe 84. I am alone and sad because I am alone. Nobody with me...."*

BC: *"Have you heard from your husband you were running away from?"*

Diane: *"No, he died a long time ago. Somebody told me that he was dead. I never saw him after leaving him."*

BC: *"Let's look back at your life as Amy. How was your life?"*

Diane: *"Very sad. I had no love. I didn't love my husband. He was a bad man. I loved my baby, but she died."*

BC: *" Was your baby girl somebody you know in the current life?"*

Diane: *"Yes, my baby was my best friend in the present life. Yes, same person. I have to die now. I am very old."*

I knew that her soul left the body. After less than a minute of silence, she started speaking again.

Diane: *"I am a man. My name is Dimitry and I am 32 years old."*

BC: *"Do you have a family of your own?"*

Diane: *"Yes, I have a wife. She is not a good woman. I don't have any feelings for her."*

BC: *"Why did you marry her?"*

Diane: *"My father said I had to. She was rich!"*

BC: *"That's fine. Do you know what year it is?"*

Diane: *"Yes, it's 1826, somewhere in Europe. I live in a nice house. My wife cannot have children."*

Instead of recalling more memories from that lifetime as Dimitry, Diane jumped quickly in another body.

Diane: *"I am in Ireland. It's 1859. I am a man and my name is James."*

BC: *"Tell me more about yourself. What do you do for a living?"*

Diane: *"I am a teacher. I teach English. Not children, just adults."*

BC: *"Are you married?"*

Diane: *"Yes. My wife is a good woman. We have two children, a boy George and a girl Cynthia. I am very proud of them."*

BC: *"Are you happy?"*

Diane: *"Very. We have a house on a hill. Happy family."*

BC: *"Where are you at the moment?"*

Diane: *"I am outside. It's raining. I am going to feed the horses. We have such a beautiful property!"*

BC: *"Do you have any other family living with you?"*

Diane: *"Yes, a brother, but I don't know his name."*

BC: *"Let's go further in time as James as I count from five to one. 5, 4, 3, 2, 1.... What do you see, hear or feel?"*

Diane: *"I am 47 now."*

BC: *"Where are your wife and children?"*

Diane: *"My wife died. She was a good wife. She was sick and died. My children are away. I don't hear too much from them. They live with their partners."*

BC: *"Do you have a new wife or are you single?"*

Diane: *"No other woman in my life."*

BC: *"That's fine. Let's now go to the very last moments in the lifetime as James. Where are you?"*

Diane: *"I am 72. I am in my house. It's a beautiful house."*

BC: *" Are you still single?"*

Diane: *"No. I have a new partner. She is a good woman. Her hair is long and plaited. She is a good wife. Her name is Cyndi."*

BC: *"Do you love her?"*

Diane: *"More than she knows."*

BC: *"Do you recognize her as being a person in the present lifetime?"*

Diane: *"Yes, she is one of my friends... a young friend."*

BC: *"Looking back to your life as James, how was that lifetime?"*

Diane: *"Very happy. I was loved. I had children. Very happy."*

After the regression session, I had a long chat with Diane. Her mood changed suddenly. Her life as James proved to her that she could be happy as she already was in other existences.

Diane left relieved. I felt that a weight was lifted from her shoulders. I then realized that, before being regressed, she believed that she didn't deserve to be happy because she may have done something really bad in another life and a curse was chasing her in the present. She was pleasantly surprised to remember how happy she was and what a beautiful life she had as James, who lived in a desirable house on the hill.

I haven't seen Diane since the regression. I often wonder if her life has changed and if she started believing in herself. Happiness starts with us believing!

I often remember Diane, mostly because I haven't had many clients mentioning a possible curse. To be perfectly honest, I don't believe in any form of curse. For me, this sounds like a Hollywood theme. However, I have to admit that a curse is just a negative thought, opposite to the positivity suggested by the Law of Attraction.

You may ask yourself what is this law I mention so often? Well, this concept is based on the fact that positive attracts positive. Therefore the Law of Attraction suggests changing your own way of thinking in order to receive, according to your wishes. Positivity is common sense by the way!

I have come across many people who swear by the Law of Attraction. I too am a believer. However I have never met a person who was certain that dark spells work. I am not saying that they wouldn't; I am saying that I don't believe in them. In my opinion, a curse is just a form of superstition.

You may have heard about the *"pharaohs curse"*, a

curse that apparently affected those who disturbed the sarcophagi of famous Egyptian pharaohs, which, by the way, was confirmed to be just a legend. Or perhaps you came across a piece of jewelry called *"the evil eye"*, which was quite popular a few centuries ago. The folklore says that this piece brings bad luck, but again I doubt that it works. What I believe however is that it is not the curse that may install fear or even destroy a life; it is the placebo effect that starts once one thinks that a spell has been cast.

LINEAR VERSUS NON-LINEAR TIME

"Time is eternity that sees its own implementations"

Plato

Most of my clients so far were able to recall with clarity months or even years of their past reincarnations. However, a few of them were confused when remembering events from two different lives that showed an overlap of time. They thought that they couldn't have been in two places at the same time. To understand this phenomenon, we should look into time as one of the properties of our Universe. Let's start with the fact that time can be defined by its own measurement.

We modern humans expect hours, days, years, decades and centuries to follow one after another in a very linear and chronological order. It is easier for our brains to perceive a linear time when moving from the past to the present and then to the future in a perfect straight line. But is time really linear? According to ancient Greek philosophers, a cyclical characteristic makes time infinite, therefore endless. Quantum physics admits the possibility of time being non-linear. Just imagine how confusing that would be for the human brain witnessing past, present and future simultaneously... or being able to travel back into the past. Past life regression makes this possible, doesn't it?

If time is non-linear, the present is where our focus is; therefore an overlap of time can be explained by moving our focus from one sequence to another. From the soul's perspective only, an incarnation may not necessarily be followed immediately by another one; the two of them may happen in a non-linear way. In other words, life is not always instantly followed by another life; it may happen in the same instance. For a better understanding, just picture yourself folding a towel. You know the length of the towel, but once folded, parts of it overlap forming pockets.

If time is defined as the point where a soul focuses its attention, then the overlap of time is more than possible. This doesn't necessarily mean that two existences happen simultaneously, but a pocket of time or an overlap of time would explain the occurrence of déjà vu. This is just a feeling of familiarity experienced by most, if not all, of us. There are people we meet who seem familiar to us and provoke the feeling that we already know them; or perhaps places that we sense as having visited before.

It may be difficult and confusing to admit that time may overlap and that one may have lived for a few years in so-called parallel lives, but I simply cannot deny this possibility. I have had clients who recalled similar experiences. Alma was one of them.

Alma is a very smart lady. In her early 50s, she is an accomplished, well-known woman. Her brain works like a computer, making her able to accumulate high quantities of information. There is no subject that would intimidate Alma. On top of that, she is a beautiful woman, taking care of herself in a way that many 21st Century women don't. Just a pleasure having her in my practice!

You may ask yourself, what brought her to my practice? Curiosity and the desire to know more about her soul.

It was on a Friday afternoon when Alma started her journey in one of her past lives.

Alma: *"I am on top of a hill. Oh, I am so beautiful! I wear beautiful Kashmir trousers that end above my ankles and a short coat. The fabric is so soft and expensive. My*

54

blouse is white silk. I wear pearls and pearl drop earrings. There is something special about me."

BC: *"Why do you think that is?"*

Alma: *"I am very well put together and stunningly beautiful.... that old-style beauty. My skin is like porcelain and my eyes are light green. I wear make-up. My hair was just styled for sure. I wear it very short at the back and I have a long fringe. My hair is black and straight. I am so familiar and comfortable in this body. I may be either wealthy or famous."*

BC: *"What else do you see? What are you doing on that hill?"*

Alma: *"I am on top of the hill sitting under a tree. There is only one tree. The sun is going down and it's almost dark. In front of me is a big city and I see many lights. It's Los Angeles no doubt. I know that I don't live there. I have a nice house in New York, but I came here for work. We are shooting."*

BC: *"Shooting?"*

Alma: *"Yes, I am an actress in silent movies. People know me."*

Alma divulged her name. For me it meant nothing, but after the session, doing a little research, I realized that the person she referred to existed. For privacy reasons, I will not make her name public.

BC: *"How old are you?"*

Alma: *"I am 32. I've been in five movies, I am good at what I do, people love me, but I believe that my career is almost over."*

BC: *"Why is that?"*

Alma: *"I will get married very soon. He is good to me. Neither of us wants children. We have all we need together: a great house and money. He gave me this brooch."*

BC: *"What brooch?"*

Alma: *"I am wearing it. It's a swan made out of little diamonds. It's beautiful. He is wealthy and spoils me."*

BC: *"Do you love him?"*

Alma: *"He is good for me. I loved somebody else, but he left me. This man treats me right. I will get married soon."*

I helped Alma travel forward in time. To be honest, I was curious to know if she married that man and if she was happy.

Alma: *"I am 54. I am still very beautiful. I take good care of myself."*

BC: *"Are you married?"*

Alma: *"My husband died. That's fine. I can live alone. I don't want another man. He was a good man. I inherited everything. He left me everything."*

BC: *"Do you still have the brooch?"*

Alma: *"I wear it every day. People now know more about my brooch than about me."*

Later in the session, Alma talked about her death.

Alma: *"It's 1980. I am old now. My skin is still beautiful. I lived a good life. I had a career, I was married, I was beautiful, people wanted me, and I had everything I wanted."*

She then told me about her experience in the life between lives.

Alma: *"There is somebody with me, but I don't see who. It's a man's voice. I believe that it may be a spirit or an angel perhaps. He doesn't speak my language, but I understand him. It's like a voice in my head. He says that happiness comes in many forms. This was my lesson: another form of happiness. I was so happy with what I was given. The voice I hear is so calm. This is because I learnt the lesson and I lived according to my destiny."*

After the regression, Alma seemed confused.

Alma: *"I don't understand. I was born in 1962. How was it possible to live two lives in the same time? I was 18 when me as an actress died."*

In her past life regression, Alma experienced a time relapse. If you ask yourself if this could actually happen in real life, just remember that Einstein believed that time is relative and flexible. According to quantum mechanics, time relapse could happen only if time is non-linear; a concept traditional physicists may or may not agree upon. However, just imagine how amazing a non-linear time could be: a form of time that creates relapses. You may be able to be in the present whilst looking or even traveling in the past and, why not, into the future. As an analogy, just imagine being on the Equator line that may represent your present. You could easily turn your head and look at the Northern Hemisphere, which for this analogy would be your past; then at the Southern Hemisphere that may be your future.

Returning to Alma's regression, what is interesting about it resides in the similarities between her life as Alma and her life as a silent movie actress. Alma's father was an architect and her mother an opera singer. So were the actress'. Alma's husband had the same birthday as her previous incarnation's husband. Were these simple coincidences or rather part of a universal code of souls? Do souls leave clues in the hope of being recognized? I am not sure that I can answer these questions, but I know that I have encountered similarities in many of the past life regressions I have conducted. The concept that the soul leaves the same fingerprint in each of its lives by following identical patterns is a tempting one. Would it be possible for a soul to be part of a purely mathematical code, whilst the clues are nothing other than symbols and numbers?

I often thought that this code may perhaps look similar to the *"Flower of Life"*, a geometric shape formed by overlapping evenly spaced and shaped circles. Each circle is in fact a pattern and each pattern is identical. However, with a closer look, the patterns seem to be changing. It may only be a visual illusion or a proof of hidden shapes. In essence, this is what makes the *"Flower of Life"* so beautiful, and quite controversial too.

Alma came back for another past life regression the next Friday evening. She expressly booked her appointment for a late time because she wanted to sleep on it and think more about the experience in her days off. I sometimes find that a few days after a regression, my clients remember more details about the past lives they were regressed to. It seems to me that new information still flows for at least two or three days after a past life regression.

Alma quickly fell into a deep hypnotic trance and

when I asked her what she recollected, she started talking. Words came out of her mouth one after another.

Alma: *"I am 18. I have very long black hair and olive skin. My eyes are dark brown. I wear a long beige dress. It's very see-through and I can see my skin underneath."*

BC: *"Where are you?"*

Alma: *"I see mountains and a kind of forest. I am outside of the forest. The mountain starts right behind the trees. It may be somewhere in South America."*

BC: *"Do you remember the year?"*

Alma: *"Long time ago. Maybe 1200."*

BC: *"Are there any people near you?"*

Alma: *"Many. There is a man in front of me who gives me a drink. It has a bitter taste. I know that I have to drink it."*

BC: *"Why is that?"*

Alma: *"I have no clue why, but I know I have to drink it. I am dizzy and so relaxed. Everything is moving. People take me somewhere, but I don't care. I see a hole in the ground. Somebody is buried there.... they want me buried with that person.... a man... an old man. They make me jump in the hole. I see people throwing soil over me. I don't fight back. I feel relaxed. I see people looking down at me."*

BC: *"Do you recognize anybody?"*

Alma: *"I don't think so. Maybe one. My neighbor."* Alma recalled dying by being buried alive. After the session, Alma said that the memories were so vivid and death was very traumatic. Her second session took her back to a lifetime, which was very different to the one she recalled in her first past life regression. One soul, two different destinies!

CHANGING DESTINY

"It is not in the stars to hold our destiny but in ourselves"

William Shakespeare

Lessons we are supposed to learn in a lifetime and the destiny within one existence are different aims of a soul. Picture your karmic lesson as being the mission statement of a business and the destiny being the business plan.

Soul decides which lesson it wants to accomplish in an existence before incarnating. If the lesson is fully understood and accomplished in the same time, the soul evolves and more than likely reincarnates to achieve another goal. On the other hand, if we fail to learn the lesson, which we signed up for, we may repeat that lesson until it is completed. In my experience, this is not set in stone. There is a possibility of making some changes to the lesson itself.

Most people seem to be interested in their destiny rather than in the karmic lessons they have to learn in their present life. This is probably because we want to make sure that we take full advantage of our abilities and potential in order to achieve as much as possible. It is only human to aim for excellence in the pursuit of accumulating as much as we can intellectually, emotionally, psychically and materially. We usually want more than we can achieve or obtain. Therefore, we believe that once we know why we are here, we can move more easily in life.

Most people believe that destiny and fate have the same meaning. However I believe that destiny is the sum of our talents or gifts, which helps us to choose one life path over another. On the other hand, I believe that fate is an effect of not following our destiny; therefore it may have a slightly negative connotation.

Just imagine yourself having the potential to become a sculptor for instance. Picture yourself naturally gifted, putting hard work into your art, studying at university everything related to possible techniques in sculpting, and having the money to organize a nice studio and to buy every sort of clay in the world. Also imagine yourself not following that path, surprising every art gallery curator who believed in you. They may say that you haven't followed your destiny. I would say that fate is what comes after that.

Some people believe that destiny is predetermined, others that fate is predestined. In the ancient world, things were clearer. For Romans, three goddesses, Athropos, Clotho and Lachesis, also called *"The Three Fates"*, were believed to predestine one's life path.

Perhaps looking at the essence of destiny and fate by establishing their etymology may give clearer answers as to what the difference between the two is. The word destiny has its origin in the Latin *"destinare"*, which means *"establish, make firm"*. This already gives an idea of the true meaning of destiny, which for me is our life's destination. On the other hand, fate comes from *"fatum"*, which in Latin means *"that which has been spoken"*; therefore the repercussions of not following your own destiny seem to be predestined or at least already agreed on.

When we refer to destiny, most people don't understand that we have free will and - even if there may be a possibility that our destiny is predetermined and agreed on by us, before coming back to life - we can make changes according to our circumstances. Our free will guarantees that.

Just imagine going to a fortuneteller to find out whether or not to accept a new job. You heard that this job was advertised; you know that they want you and that they have even offered the position to you, so all you want to clarify is whether or not this job is part of your destiny. Now imagine that the reader tells you to go for it because you are meant to have that job. From this point here, to quitting your existing job and accepting that particular new one, is another story. You have free will. You can accept the job or decline it, no matter what the fortuneteller predicted earlier. In each of your actions, you have at least two choices: yes or no. There is a third choice by the way: yes, but *"not just yet"* or *"no for now"*. Therefore, even if your soul may have decided and agreed upon a destiny, or not, there is always a point where you can make some changes to it or even follow a completely different path.

Once you know that you can use the power of your free will in following your karmic lesson and your destiny, you may ask yourself what exactly is predestined and cannot be changed. Well, I believe that meeting some people is inevitable. I also believe that your soul and theirs have signed an agreement before reincarnating to interfere in each other's lives. No matter whether these connections impact your life in a positive or negative way, you still learn and evolve from these relationships.

I believe that one cannot avoid meeting their twin soul. Twin souls are controversial subjects. Some believe that we all have one somewhere, others don't. Twin souls are mirrors of our souls and have been formed by our own soul's division. I am skeptical about the fact that twin souls are always reincarnated at the same time, therefore in the same lifetime. I am also not convinced that a relationship with a twin soul is like a breeze, but if it becomes like that then your soul feels complete. Usually a meeting of twin souls helps them both evolve, mainly on a spiritual level. I don't deny the fact that romantic love can be involved, but at a purely spiritual level, each unconsciously encourages the other to develop. I would say that meeting your twin soul could be both a blessing... and a curse too; it depends on the level of development that each has already achieved.

Many of my clients believe that their love partners are their twin souls. Most of them have been intrigued that they haven't recalled any memories of these so called *"flame souls"* in any of the regressions they had. To be honest, presumptions of a past life regression may not meet the client's expectations. In my experience, many clients hope to recall lives in which they have been famous, on top of the world, happy, loved and wealthy. The truth may be totally different.

If twin souls are controversial subjects, the story about soulmates is straightforward. A soulmate doesn't necessarily have to be a lover or a life partner. Some people believe their pets are their soulmates and they may well be so. Others that their teachers or gurus are their soulmates. Who says this cannot happen? One thing is certain: it is the soul's duty to find other souls it has to connect with, also the soul's privilege to learn from each soul it interacts with.

IN AND OUT OF LIVES

"I did not begin when I was born, nor when I was conceived"

Jack London

If you believe in reincarnation, your theory about it may sound like this: we were born, we die, then born and die again and so on life after life; same soul, a destiny and a lesson for each life. At least this was my understanding a long time ago. It sounds simple and so plausible. Let me just tell you that things may be a little bit more complicated. I have witnessed past life regressions where my clients stepped in and out of lives. Just like that! They recalled memories from a previous lifetime and, at some stage, they jumped into another existence and then returned back to the initial one... or not.

Do existences happen simultaneously based on the theory of the time being non-linear or is life followed by life in a straight timeline? Or perhaps a relapse of a certain period of time may happen in a particular past life? And, if this was just a pocket of time, was stepping out of an existence necessary in order to achieve a lesson or a life path? Does stepping back into a previous lifetime for a similar purpose mean that the lesson in that existence could have been avoided, as it was already learnt in another parallel or not existence? I am not sure whether there is one single person on this planet who can argue that they have a precise answer for all of these questions. We all make suppositions based on our beliefs or what we were taught.

However, what I know for sure is that I have witnessed clients stepping out of a lifetime, stepping into another one and then back again. I don't believe that their memories got confused. I rather suspect that a jump from one existence to another may have been absolutely necessary from the karmic lesson's perspective. What better example than Karen?

Karen is a beautiful young lady. She lives in another town, three hours away from my practice. I was surprised when she called and booked a regression as I knew there was some travel involved, but she was stubborn. Karen said that she heard about me from one of her friends and she thought that a regression was her last resort, to find out if bad karma from a past existence was following her. She had a suspicion that she may have experienced this current life before, or at least something very similar to her present existence.

She arrived on a Friday afternoon and, once I met her, I knew that I already liked her. She told me that she recently left a bad relationship, but all she could think about was her ex-partner. Not that she wanted him back. She just wanted to see him punished, for leaving her for one of her friends.

Karen explained that her relationship had seemed stable enough to buy a house together. They wanted children and started trying for a family. After the break, they had to sell their house and she was left with almost nothing. Therefore she blamed her current situation on her ex-partner and she was convinced that she hated him. Karen couldn't help herself constantly checking if he was happy or not, while really wishing that he was utterly unhappy.

I sympathized with her mostly because I had the feeling that I really understood her: she was honest, loyal, very beautiful…. and she deserved the best. Just a very pleasant person!

Karen let herself go into a deep trance and, whilst relaxed, she seemed even more beautiful.

BC: *"Where are you?"*

Karen: *"I see the ocean. There are waves... big waves. They are noisy.... waves' noise."*

BC: *"Do you recognize the place? Have you been there before?"*

Karen: *"No, it's a different ocean. I never saw it before. It is very dark, but I know that I am in the middle of the ocean.... on a boat.... very big boat, but I cannot see what boat. Very big boat..."*

BC: *"Are there any people around you?"*

Karen: *"I'm alone.... and it's so dark and I hear the noises the waves make."*

BC: *"Now, look down to your feet. Are they bigger or smaller, or maybe different? What are you wearing, sandals, boots, animal skin or perhaps do you have bare feet?"*

Karen: *"I cannot see them. It's so dark. I know that I am a woman.... older woman.... much older. It's so dark and scary. I feel uncomfortable."*

BC: *"That's fine. Nothing can harm you. Do you know what year it is?"*

71

Karen: *"Yes. It's 1509. I am on that boat in the middle of the ocean.... in between lands. It's very wet. My feet are wet.... and my clothes too... and it's dark, very dark, and scary."*

BC: *"What are you doing on that boat?"*

Karen: *"I don't know. I am alone. Something must have happened. I may not be alone after all.... I think that there may be somebody else on the boat.... close to me. I am very wet."*

BC: *"Tell me what happens."*

Karen: *"I bend down. Water. Hmmm.... maybe I....."*

BC: *"Maybe what?"*

I waited for Karen to answer and I was surprised when she did. I expected her to carry on remembering her life as an old woman on a boat in the middle of the ocean. But instead, she stepped out of that lifetime and stepped into another existence.

Karen: *"I am in a church. It's daylight and there is so much white around me. There are many people in the church."*

BC*: "Do you know where this church may be?"*

Karen: *"I am in the UK... country church... maybe in a village."*

I realized that she was not an old woman anymore. The scene has changed as she stepped into another lifetime.

BC: *"Look down to your feet or perhaps to your clothes. What are you wearing?"*

Karen: *"A nice white dress. It's very nice and soft. People like it."*

BC: *"Are you a bride?"*

Karen: *"Yes, I am. I am young. Oh.... it's my wedding day."*

BC: *"How old are you?"*

Karen: *"27.... Yes, I am 27 years old."*

BC: *"Look at the people around you. Do you recognize any of them as being part of your present life?"*

Karen: *"Yes, my brother is here. I recognize my brother. He is happy."*

The person Karen recognized was her brother in her present life.

BC: *"And you? Are you happy?"*

Karen: *"Very happy. It's my wedding day. I am getting married today. I wear a long white dress. I have long hair."*

BC: *"Do you see your husband to be?"*

Karen: *"He is not here yet. I am waiting. His name is Max. I love him heaps. I am so happy. Yes, very happy."*

BC: *"So it's a happy memory..."*

Karen: *"Very happy. White dress...."*

BC: *"Has the groom arrived?"*

Karen: *"No. I am still waiting. I am not scared. He will come... but he hasn't yet."*

BC: *"Look around you again. Do you recognize anybody else whilst waiting?"*

Karen: *"Just my brother.... Max is still not here. He will come...."*

Karen started being anxious, so I decided to move her a few minutes further in time. And again she stepped out of that past life and stepped into a totally different person.

Karen: *"I am walking. I see trees. I think I am in a forest."*

BC: *"How old are you?"*

Karen: *"Not that old. I am a young woman. Not very old... maybe the same."*

BC: *"Why are you walking? Where are you going?"*

Karen: *"Not sure... just walking. I see trees."*

BC: *"What happens?"*

Karen: *"Something crashes. I hear the noise... maybe a branch or a tree. I think it falls on me."*

BC: *"What else?"*

Karen: *"I don't feel any pain. Something landed on me... like it's over."*

BC: *"Tell me what do you see or feel."*

Karen: *"Clouds."*

BC: *"What else?"*

Instead of continuing with her story, Karen stepped back into her body as a bride.

Karen: *"I don't think Max is coming. I stopped hoping. I left the church."*

BC: *"Take your time. Do you know what your lesson in that lifetime may have been?"*

Karen: *"Love and trust.... and laughter."*

After the regression Karen confessed that the lesson she mentioned was in fact related to the lifetime as a young woman just about to get married. She said that she already knew that her groom would not come. She also realized that she would be left alone at the altar. She had the feeling that she ran away into a forest, but when she tried to remember what happened next, she jumped into a similar scene from a different lifetime. Therefore, she saw herself dying in a forest under the weight of a tree. She assumed that perhaps something similar had happened to her after she left the altar, or at least both deaths may have had something in common.

She also said she had the feeling that, in the first lifetime she recalled, she bent over and fell into the water, but she knew that her mind refused to remember this. She tried hard to block that memory.

UNRESOLVED BUSINESS IN A PAST LIFE

"No excellent soul is exempt from a mixture of madness"

Aristotle

There is a common belief that everything we experience on a physical or emotional level in a lifetime finishes once death occurs. This may be the case for some. How would you then argue unexplained phobias that have absolutely no obvious origin in the present?

We are not born with phobias. The only fears we have at birth are the fear of falling and the fear of loud noises. It is said that phobias are learnt over time. I totally agree that this is the case, but what if some phobias are carried from one life to another in the same manner we could inherit promises, contracts or even feelings from one existence to another? It is really debatable which emotions are caused by our own ego and which are triggered from other lifetimes.

For example, just picture that you borrow money from an old friend without discussing a contract. Also imagine that a week before you are due to make the repayment, your friend dies and there is no successor to whom you can repay the debt. Some would think this was your good fortune, but most would struggle with the idea that they owe money with no way of repaying it. This feeling would make them less free, more indebted and may even haunt them. A promise made in a past life could carry on in a very similar way. It is unresolved business that triggers other unpleasant emotions in the present.

There is a possibility that some phobias, anchored in a past existence, may distress you in the present life exactly as unresolved businesses can. In certain circumstances, this could trigger particular behavior in the current lifetime. I witnessed this phenomenon with many clients. Victoria was one of them. I regressed her a year after I met her.

Victoria is a gorgeous looking woman. In her early 30s, she has a perfect face, beautiful hazel green eyes and a personality to die for. Victoria is bubbly and fun and everybody loves her. When I met her, she had a successful home hairdressing salon and didn't struggle to get new clients. As I've said, everybody loved her. However her dreams were far greater than being just a hairdresser - not that she wasn't an excellent one.

When I met her, just a year ago, Victoria was a spiritual being and recently became an energy practitioner in one of the therapy fields that have become popular in recent years. She dreamt of putting her hairdressing career behind her, but she feared that she wouldn't be able to make enough money. Victoria's husband was a lovely young guy who had a good job, but her income was still needed to contribute to the bills and the upbringing of her two children. She feared not being able to build up her new business to the same level as her hairdressing. Her main concern however was that she lacked the knowledge, and that she may be too young to be taken seriously. Victoria had in-built fears. She delayed and postponed the decision day after day, which, to be honest, made her very unhappy.

Despite the 20 year gap between us, Victoria and I became friends and one day I offered to do a past life regression for her. I explained that there was a possibility this fear of *"everything and nothing"* may have come from one of her past lives. Maybe she thought to herself that, if this therapy cannot help, at least it cannot do any harm. So one Tuesday around lunchtime she arrived at my practice, bubbly and fun as always.

We chatted for a little while and I thought to myself that this young woman is so gifted.... if she only knew that! Neither of us knew at that stage that, right after the session, Victoria's future would turn out exactly the way she hoped.

Victoria: *"I see a big manor house. There is a large lawn around it and horses. It is a very appealing property."*

BC: *"That's nice. What are you wearing?"*

Victoria: *"I wear a long brown dress.... a beautiful dress with some patterns... maybe lines. It's beautiful. I am a young girl, maybe 16. I have long hair and brown eyes. My name is Madeleine. I have the feeling that I am very happy. I think that we are quite wealthy."*

BC: *"Do you know what year it is?"*

Victoria: *"Definitely. It's 1872. I am in Europe. Switzerland is the country."*

BC: *"Do you have any family?"*

Victoria: *"Yes, I have a mother and a father. They are both inside doing something. I am outside on the lawn. I have a four year old sister. I think that her name is Anna or something very similar. I don't have a boyfriend. I don't really know many boys around my age."*

BC: *"So what are you doing outside?"*

Victoria: *"Just resting. I am sick. I cough a lot and my parents called the doctor."*

BC: *"What else is happening?"*

Victoria: *"The doctor must have arrived because I am now on my bed, inside. I look very grey and cough a lot. It's a serious illness."*

Victoria started coughing and I realized that her soul would leave her body very shortly. And it did.

Victoria: *"I died young.... just 16, but I had a good life. I was well looked after, and my parents loved me. We were wealthy and had everything we wanted. I had nice dresses. I was out in nature every day. It's just the illness that wasn't nice."*

BC: *"Can you recall what your soul learnt in that lifetime?"*

Victoria: *"Family! I learnt how important family was!"*

A few minutes later, Victoria's soul found a new body in a totally different existence.

Victoria: *"I am a boy. My hair is very blond. We are poor and live in a box house. It's very tiny."*

BC: *"Tell me about your family."*

Victoria: *"I have a baby sister… she's very young… and parents. Life is so hard for us all."*

BC: *"Do you know where you are?"*

Victoria: *"It's Germany. I am too young to know the year. I wear brown, rough trousers. There is a radio in the small kitchen and I hear the music. I think that I am sick."*

Before asking her more questions, the little boy experienced death. Then Victoria jumped straight into another lifetime.

Victoria: *"I am a 19 year old girl. My name sounds something like Yvonne. It's like a war or something because I hear the guns. I don't know why, but I had to go outside.... maybe to bring something in. I am afraid that I would die."*

BC: *"What do you see, hear or feel?"*

Victoria: *"They shot me I guess because I fell down and I feel the pain."*

Another few minutes later, she started talking again.

Victoria: *"Angels are taking me under their wings. They heal me. They tell me that sometimes you cannot control your life. Most times you cannot control your death. Sometimes you have to die young. Life is short... it goes so fast. Always follow your gut, they say. If you live your life in honesty, everything is possible. Pure love and gratitude for what you have... just pure love."*

After the regression, it was clear to me that Victoria's fear of not being good enough may have been caused in the lives she had recalled. In each of them, happy or sad, poor or rich, boy or girl, she died young, not being allowed to develop, grow and to achieve something. Perhaps her only current fear was that the present life wouldn't allow her dream to develop because she was too young to dare to reach for the stars.

Time passed, and a month later, Victoria closed her hairdressing salon, and then opened her new practice. Her skills and determination brought her the immediate success that she deserved on her new journey. She transformed into a wonderful butterfly!

Time has passed since Victoria's regression and many things have changed. Victoria has no fear of the future. Meanwhile, our friendship has grown and, being two Virgos, Victoria and I even taught several workshops together; and we have others planned for the future.

Victoria's regression makes me believe that sometimes healing has to begin back in our distant past, in another time, perhaps in a past life. In my opinion, experiencing death again after a life that has triggered unwanted problems might heal your soul. On top of that, the doors of those lives may close properly and the door to success may open in the present life. Because when one door closes, another one opens.

WE ARE HERE TO LEARN A LESSON

"The greatest blessings of mankind are within us and within our reach."

Seneca

Many people cannot imagine themselves in a different habitat than in the one they currently reside. The language they speak, the area they live, their family, social connections and daily circumstances are all they know. And this is perfectly normal. We were born into an environment that comprises our whole existence. We then develop our own bubble of individuality, based on traditional beliefs mixed with our own experiences. However, the universal picture is much bigger. I usually tell people that the Universe doesn't speak English; it speaks in vibrations, in that special way that everybody all over the world can understand the whole truth.

Sometimes we perceive ourselves as being average and very small in comparison to the universal consciousness. We are all average and spectacular at the same time. We all belong to souls that, with each existence, become closer to perfection. We are all a work in progress, some less developed, others on higher levels. The beauty of life is that we do not have a clue which is which. Behind your neighbor, who seems so average, may be a soul that has learnt much more than you. Or the other way around!

We sometimes feel proud and hold our heads high because we believe we live a better life than others, without showing any compassion or empathy for our less fortunate fellow humans.

Just because we are wealthy and health doesn't mean that our karma is immaculate, and our souls are just about to reach Nirvana. Just because we drive an expensive and fast sports car and live in a mansion doesn't make us more evolved than others. Remember that, at the soul level, we all have lessons to learn and maybe our lesson is abundance. Who says that our poor neighbor's lesson is not abundance too? He, the neighbor, may be barely able to feed his children, doesn't own a car or a house, but he may have decided to learn the same lesson from a different approach.

We are all different and so alike too. Some of us are visual, others audio, kinesthetic or audiovisual, and so are the perspectives of a lesson. We can approach it from different angles. Our truth is subjective and not always shared by others: the truth is what you believe in as an individual. The fact is, we have lived all around the world according to our circumstances in past lives, perhaps very differently from how we conduct things in our present life. Past life regression definitely proves that!

A person who understood this was Kaya. She booked a past life regression purely out of curiosity. From the first moment I met her, she said that she was open to anything and everything. She wanted to know and she wanted to learn.

Kaya is a delicate woman in her early 50s. She lives in a beautiful house, in a perfect neighborhood, drives a desirable car, and has an amazing job and a loyal and loving husband. Everything about her seems perfect.

When I first met Kaya, I noticed that she was beautiful but thought to myself that she was even more beautiful than she knew because she was empathetic, compassionate, gentle and very humble.

Her session was late on a Thursday evening after

she finished work. She wore color-coordinated clothes and looked immaculate. We built a rapport very quickly and I knew that she trusted the whole process... and me. Therefore, she allowed herself to get hypnotized very quickly.

Kaya: *"I am on a field, digging holes in the ground. I think I'm planting something. There are around twenty people planting too. I see a wagon very close to me. Maybe it transported us to the field."*

BC: *"Do you know what year it is?"*

Kaya: *"It's 1842.... or 1843. I am Irish but live somewhere else. I emigrated to a new land."*

BC: *"Are you a woman or a man?"*

Kaya: *"I am a woman. I have long brown, very thick hair. I am just young. It's so hot in the field and I am sweaty."*

BC: *"Where is your family, if you have any?"*

Kaya: *"I am not sure whether my parents are still alive or not. I left them when I left my country, Ireland. My husband died. I have two young boys, but they are not with me. I work very hard... very, very hard."*

BC: *"What language are the people around you speaking?"*

Kaya: *"It's not English. I don't understand what*

they are saying. They are talking weird."

BC: *"Do you remember why you left your country?"*

Kaya: *"I came on a boat. My husband and I wanted to make a new life for us. We were poor in Ireland. We came to this island for a better life, but my husband died. I have to work for my children."*

BC: *"Where are they now?"*

Kaya: *"I left them with an old woman in the village. She looks after them while I work. Money is not enough.... we would go back to Ireland, but money is not enough. I don't have enough to live and not enough to go back to Ireland."*

BC: *"How do you make yourself understood if you don't speak the language?"*

Kaya: *"There is a man who's helping me. He knows this language. His name is Dennis. He came from Ireland too, but he learnt the language. He translates."*

I decided to take Kaya to her death scene and, knowing what a hard life she had, I wondered when that might have happened.

Kaya: *"I am not very old. Just before 40. I am heavily pregnant and alone. I think that I am in a forest."*

BC: *"What are you doing in the forest?"*

Kaya: *"I am giving birth to a new baby. The father is the man who translates for me. He left us and left the village. I haven't heard from him since. I am in the forest that every maid or poor girl goes to, to give birth. It's a shame. I am not married. The child has no father."*

BC: *"Tell me what happens."*

Kaya: *"The baby is not coming. I am full of blood and in pain. Maybe the baby is dead inside me.... yes, the baby is dead. I am not feeling well. I have high temperature and there is blood everywhere."*

Kaya died trying to give birth to her baby. I let her rest for a few minutes then asked her where she was.

Kaya: *"I am home. It's so bright, just full of light. I feel so happy and healed. I know that my baby should be here somewhere.... healing too. I hear a voice saying that next time I should not be fooled. My lesson in this life was trust. The voice says that everything is fine."*

After the session, we had a long chat. I usually allocate time after every session to discuss the experiences my clients recalled in past lives and how they could positively affect their present life. I want to make sure that my clients understand what has just happened and that they are comfortable and able to talk openly about the whole experience. You cannot change the past; this is always the main lesson.

Kaya had tears in her eyes. She sympathized with the woman she was and was sorry for her suffering. She said that she had the feeling that she was on a Polynesian island and couldn't understand why she and her husband emigrated there. *"We must have been very desperate"*, she said.

She then opened up more and told me that she had started working with unfortunate people and, from the first day in her new job, despite her wealth, she felt that she was one of them.

I thought about Kaya for a long time after her regression. She proved to me that somewhere deep in our hearts, we remember. We do things in our present lives that may be based on what we have done in another life. We may feel empathy for people we knew hundreds of years ago. It is only a matter of recognizing that and trusting our intuition.

DEJA VU

"The secret of change is to focus all of your energy not on fighting the old, but on building the new."

Socrates

Usually my clients ring or email to book appointments. None of them pop in to secure their therapy sessions because I don't have a secretary. My mobile is usually on silent, so, at the end of each day, I listen to my messages and get in touch with potential clients. I give everybody the same attention.

I remember very well one specific evening. It was cold and rainy, as winter evenings in New Zealand usually are, and I was so looking forward to lighting a fire, having dinner and relaxing whilst watching an episode of my favorite TV series. It was a Friday evening after a week full of clients. I had already listened to my messages, contacted clients back and made all the bookings for the next weeks.

I was so ready for a nice and relaxing Friday evening when my phone rang again. The lady on the other end introduced herself as Marion and asked for the earliest appointment available. I even thought that this might be a sign because the main character in my favorite TV series was also called Marion. I usually ask my clients if this is an emergency situation and, if so, I try booking them as soon as possible. So I made the booking required by Marion for the end of the following week and I went back to my usual Friday evening activities.

Marion arrived for her appointment a half an hour early. She was waiting in her car and I thought to myself that this lady was really keen. Looking out of my practice window, I noticed that Marion was a short and fragile lady in her mid 70s. She was one of my oldest clients... and as I discovered later, one of the wisest too.

We had a little introductory chat, just enough to get to know each other a little bit and to find out the motives behind her desire to be regressed. Marion told me that she had just sold the farm that she and her husband had owned for more than 40 years and bought a smaller property. From her remarks in relation to the farm, the property they bought may have been smaller, but was still huge for an older couple. The house they bought was indeed smaller, but the surrounding land was a block of a few acres, which involved regular maintenance. Marion said that her past life regression was somehow connected to this property. She had the feeling that she had lived there before. She said that aspects of the property, the trees, the river, bushes and rocks seemed to her so familiar. From the first day they moved in, she recognized everything.

Marion was born and bred in New Zealand - more specifically, in this area - so I tried convincing her that the familiarity stemmed from her knowledge of the native flora and fauna of the district. She insisted though that she had lived on the same block of land before, maybe in another life. She said that she even had reoccurring dreams about her new property and that she often had the feeling that there was an entity living in her house. This made me think that she may have been fantasizing and I just hoped that she would not be disappointed with the life she chose to travel to. So I started inducing hypnosis and hoped for the best.

BC: *"Describe what you see, hear or feel. Where are you?"*

Marion: *"I am on a ship. There are many people on the same boat. I don't see their faces very clearly, but I know that some look familiar."*

BC: *"What are you wearing?"*

Marion: *"I wear boots and a cotton dress. I don't think that my dress is a bright color... maybe grey. My hair is blond and I wear a white bonnet."*

BC: *"How old are you?"*

Marion: *"20 something... maybe 23. I am just young. People on the boat call me Janice. Yes, Janice is my name."*

BC: *"What are you doing on that boat? Where are you going?"*

Marion: *"I am on the way to a new land. My husband is on the boat too. He is organizing something with another man. I can see him talking to that man... maybe organizing something."*

BC: *"Where are you coming from and where are you going?"*

Marion: *"I am from Scotland. I was born there. We are going to New Zealand. We heard about people going there and having land. We want a better life. I am so excited, and I can't wait to arrive. Just imagine what life could be there... a house.... land..."*

BC: *"What year is it?"*

Marion: *"It's 1847. I know that because I was born*

in 1824."

BC: *"What else is happening?"*

Marion: *"It's daylight... maybe midday. My husband is still organizing something with that man. My husband is very tall and well built. There are many people traveling with us. We are all happy."*

Marion was going on and on about how hopeful and happy everybody was. She talked about the hard life back in Scotland and about the desire she had to own land. So I helped her move to another scene in that lifetime, one that she picked and one that seemed significant to that particular existence.

BC: *"Tell me what you see, hear or feel."*

Marion: *"I see land... trees, bush and... a large beach. I never saw a beach like this. Gold sand... There are people on the beach... just natives. Some have darker skin than mine. I am so happy to arrive and so pleased to be off the boat. We have to start life from scratch. We have only a few things; whatever we had back in Scotland... almost nothing. My husband carries most of our belongings."*

Marion started being excited again and even laughing. She couldn't stop talking about the flowers and the trees she was seeing on her land of opportunity. So again, I moved her to another scene in her life as Janice.

BC: *"Tell me what happens."*

Marion: *"My husband has gone somewhere. I think that he is working. I am 30 something... maybe 32. I have two daughters who are home with me. Maybe I cook something because there are many carrots on a table."*

BC: *"Do you have a house and land as you hoped?"*

Marion: *"We live in a small wooden building with an open fire. It's just small, but I like it. There is land around me... and a river... bush everywhere. When my husband works, I am in charge and that's fine. It's just that I don't feel very safe now. People are constantly fighting for land. I don't think that I am in danger, but I am so small, just petite, and I am always afraid for my daughters."*

Marion started talking about cooking and I thought to myself that she might have been a good cook in that lifetime. As I counted down from five to one, she moved to another scene in that existence.

Marion: *"I am in the same house, but many years later. There are so many houses around me now. There is even a port near us. We could have moved, but I loved this house and the land. I love this land. I know everybody who lives near me. I have friends. We all work together and help each other. I am very happy."*

BC: *"Where is your family?"*

Marion: *"My husband is working again. He always works that man. He is a good man. Our daughters are young teenagers. Good girls! They help me in the garden. We have a beautiful garden.... and land!"*

Marion as Janice lived a dream life in a dreamland. I was very curious to find out more, but I realized that I had already spent almost two hours with Marion. So I asked her to remember the last moments of that lifetime.

Marion: *"I am nearly 50. Not yet 50. My head hurts. I am ill and I am in bed."*

BC: *"Is there anybody with you?"*

Marion: *"My husband is here... our girls too. There are many of our friends with me. They are all very nice. I love them all. I don't want to leave. I don't want to die, but I am very ill. I love it here. "*

A few minutes later, Marion saw herself floating.

Marion: *"I learnt how to survive in a foreign land. And I was young when I arrived there. This is quite an accomplishment. I wanted to own land and I did. Everything happened as I wanted it to. I had a good family and many friends. Happy, happy life."*

After the regression, Marion confirmed that the

property she recalled in the past life was the property she owns in the present. Were Marion and Janice's properties at the same location? Marion believed they were. But even if they weren't, they looked very similar!

After Marion left, I spent a good half an hour thinking about what just happened, asking myself whether or not it would be possible to live more than once on the same piece of land in different lives. Then I remembered about all those stories I heard as a child of people who could recognize every street and corner in a city before witnessing it.

In a very similar way, I am sure that you have met people and asked them, or have been asked, *"have we met before?"*. Then you tried, without success, to establish, when you might have seen each other before. This is nothing other than déjà vu.

The feeling of déjà vu of a place is very similar to the strong emotion we experience when we first meet somebody we feel we have known for a long time. As I have said, déjà vu is a common feeling related to people we possibly knew in other lives. Our soul recognizes theirs even if in the present our roles may have changed. We reincarnated together because we had not finished what we were meant to complete in a past life or just because we can help each other learn the lesson we decided to focus on in the current life.

A similar phenomenon may happen with regards to a place, a country, even a continent. We feel drawn to a place we have never seen in the present life without being able to explain why. Something pulls us there because our soul knows this place; and when we finally get there, the feeling is astonishing. We may have had unfinished business in another life and felt the need to come back and finish what we started, or we returned because it was the only place we knew we would feel at home. Once there, everything seems so normal, exactly as it should be!

RELIGION VERSUS SPIRITUALITY

"Spirituality is meant to take us beyond our tribal identity
into a domain of awareness that is more universal"

Deepak Chopra

My clients have often asked me how I view spirituality. I understand their willingness to learn and their concern that they may have to believe in something else in order to "achieve" spirituality. Firstly, you don't have to believe in anything other than your natural alignment to the universal forces. You are a spiritual being. We are all created this way. Well, now I have used the word *"created"* and you may be wondering about creation versus natural selection? Don't go down that road because this question is not necessary!

Secondly, we are individuals, meant to be aware of our

own consciousness, and part of a universal conglomerate, which means we are just a little cog in the complicated global or universal consciousness' mechanism. In the same way that our soul has its own identity, it evolves because of the connections with other souls that are part of the same universal consciousness.

Many of my clients also ask if it is necessary to embrace a religion in order to reach a certain level of spirituality. I believe that religion has nothing to do with spirituality. You see, religions are mixtures of beliefs and rituals. Each religion is based on a belief that differentiates it from other religions. To be more specific, the structure of these beliefs makes a religion stand out. This would never happen in the absence of the rituals, which are sets of dogmas, mantras, symbols and so on. Let's just look at Christianity and take as example the birth of Jesus Christ. All Christians believe Jesus is the son of God. They also believe that Jesus was born at a specific time of the year, agreed to be Christmas, but they approach his birth differently. The Christmas ritual, which is the celebration itself, defines or differentiates Christian cults on Jesus' birth allegory. Same belief, different rituals that created various cults!

So, no, you don't have to be religious in order to be

spiritual, but you have to be open to understanding your mission on this planet. Each of your incarnations aims to find their role on this planet. They were all born, learnt and taught lessons and left a legacy behind. They all interacted with other human beings for that same purpose to learn and teach lessons in order to evolve and, when they found themselves back home, in the level we call *"life between lives"*, decided to come back and learn even more.

If religion has nothing to do with spirituality, what does? Well, spirituality means the awareness or recognition of something bigger than our own little lives. This cannot happen in the absence of life itself. Spirituality doesn't worship anything beyond our own understanding. So, what is bigger than us? I believe that the connection between people and the admission that we are all One defines spirituality and gives us a purpose as human beings. This happens at a personal consciousness level or state because every single experience in this life has its origin in qualia, which represents every aspect of our conscious experiences. The sum of these experiences forms our own consciousness. Our brain generates experiences and therefore our personal consciousness.

I believe that understanding consciousness involves the principles of quantum physics, and that the concept of consciousness could revolutionize science. Once science agrees what consciousness is, areas such as hypnosis, dreams, meditation and transcendence would be defined and understood more clearly. Unfortunately, at this particular moment, there is no scientific unity on defining consciousness, just as there are also no scientific tools to demystify it.

There is sometimes confusion between consciousness and conscience and I have heard many of my clients mixing these two terms. The truth is that consciousness is based on our own thoughts, feelings, beliefs, memories and environmental influences, whilst conscience is based on the sense of moral versus immoral.

Some of my clients are confused about consciousness and mindfulness. Others even believe that these two are the same. To cut a long story short, I would say that mindfulness is bringing your attention to present experiences. Mindfulness is a prominent element in Buddhism. Usually mindfulness can develop through meditation. I teach mindfulness meditation which is a guided meditation that I will discuss later.

To make the concept of consciousness easier to understand, think of it as self-awareness. If you can shift your consciousness to a higher level with increased self-awareness, a more meaningful life should unfold with ease.

As I've said, I am a spiritual person and I don't follow any of the religions. However, most of my clients, if not all, ask me my view on God. Well, for me, God is essence or energy. In this regard only, my views on a higher energy may have connotations in pantheism. I like to believe that I am not restricting myself to anything and that no dogma is part of my life. But, again, that is just me!

TAPPING INTO SPIRITUALITY

"Everything goes; everything comes back; everything rolls the wheel of being"

Nietzsche

I have had many clients who were in search of inner peace and spirituality. Some of them have just become aware of their inner world whilst stepping onto their spiritual path. This makes me think that there may be a time in all our lives when we choose awareness rather than living a life just to please others.

Once regressed into past lives, many of my clients have expressed a desire to know more about what their purpose in life is. They actually tap into spirituality. Most of them have kept in touch with me and updated me on their own progress in life. At the end of the day, we have already developed a strong connection in that special moment when I witnessed their vulnerability, whilst telling me their experiences in past lives. One of these very special clients was James.

I was in Australia visiting my son when my phone rang. All my clients knew that I was away and I even left a note about being overseas for a week on my website and my social media pages. But the phone rang, and I instantly and intuitively perceived the urgency of the person on the other end. I also realized that I have never met the person who was calling... otherwise they would have known that I was away!

I answered and heard a very joyful masculine voice. The guy introduced himself as James and asked for an appointment. I booked him for the next week. I thought that was it, but James texted me a day later to confirm the appointment.... that he had already confirmed in the first place. I understood then that he was excited to be regressed.

He arrived on a rainy Friday morning and I liked him from the first moment. In his early 40s, he was smart, happy and very curious about life in general. He had a pleasant British accent and he told me that he was born and raised somewhere in the UK, and later in life emigrated to

New Zealand. I sympathized already with him because I was an immigrant myself... also because my husband was born in the same land as James.

I always ask my clients why they want to be regressed. For James it was a matter of understanding more about his own purpose in life. James was very spiritual, so we talked about meditation, soul and karma; and a few minutes later I started inducing hypnosis.... and it was straightforward. Not long after, I began asking questions and the answers came so naturally.

James: *"I am outside. It is a beautiful day and the sky is blue. It's very hot. I think I am on top of a small building because I see the street just below me. I am looking down to the street that is empty. Nobody on the street... not far, there is a tower with a clock."*

BC: *"Look at your feet. What are you wearing?"*

James: *"I am a young boy and I wear children's shoes. My name is Thomas. I have short blonde hair and brown eyes."*

BC: *"What are you doing on top of that building?"*

James: *"I think I am on my roof. Looks like my house. I am just looking and playing."*

BC: *"What year is it?"*

James: *"I heard my parents saying that is 1920."*

BC: *"Are your parents around?"*

James: *"I don't know where they are, but not here ... maybe at work. I am alone. I am an only child and I love that. I love being alone."*

BC: *"I will now count from five to one and, as I reach one, I want you to find yourself in another scene in the lifetime as Thomas, one that has a significant message for you."*

James: *"I am 25. I am hiding, but I am not sure why. I hear a gun ... maybe a gun fight."*

BC: *"What are you wearing?"*

James: *"Green woolen jacket and boots."*

BC: *"Are there any people around you?"*

James: *"There are, but they seem to look in the opposite way. People can't see me and I want to get to them, but they can't see me. I am hiding from other people. They don't see me either."*

BC: *"But you see them. What are they wearing?"*

James: *"Uniforms .... like me. There is a man next to me. He turns to me and smiles."*

BC: *"Do you recognize him?"*

James: *"Yes, his name is George. He is young too .... just 20 years old."*

BC: *"What else happens?"*

James: *"They caught me. I am blindfolded, but I know that there is a squad in front of me. They want to shoot me. Bang...."*

I knew that his soul left his body because James became suddenly even more relaxed. I left him for a few minutes to enjoy the silence.

BC: *"Where are you now?"*

James: *"I am not sure, but it is very nice. It's silent. There are no voices, but there are vibrations and I understand them... high frequencies... vibrations. I know what they mean. They tell me you cannot do things by yourself. You need others. Vibrations.... They say that everything is fine."*

I looked at the clock on the wall and I realized that there was enough time to take James to another lifetime, if he can see himself jumping into another body. And he did because, before I was able to say anything, he already started talking.

James: *"I am in a jungle. Everything is so green. Maybe it's not a jungle, but there are trees, palms and plants all around me. The colors are so vivid."*

BC: *"Where is this jungle, do you know?"*

James: *"Yes, it's close to Perth."* (Australia)

BC: *"So what are you doing there?"*

James: *"I hunt, I have a sort of a weapon and I hunt for my family. I see my skin. I have darker skin, almost brown."*

BC: *"Your family?"*

James: *"I am married, and I have two small children, a boy and a girl. The little boy has beautiful curly hair."*

James had no children in the present life and I was not very sure that he wanted any.

BC: *"Do you remember their names?"*

James: *"I do, but I cannot pronounce them. They sound so weird. My name sounds odd too."*

BC: *"How old are you?"*

James: *"30 sharp."*

BC: *"Where do you live?"*

James:*" Oh, I live in a very lush, natural, futuristic environment. It's pretty and so organic."*

BC: *"Tell me more about your family."*

James: *"Oh, I love them so much. My wife is gorgeous. Brown skin, big eyes, soft…"*

I moved James to another time in that existence. It seemed that his whole life was flat with no big major events. He had a loving family and enjoyed living in nature. I decided to ask him to visualize his own death.

James: *"I am old. They are many people next to me. They are holding hands and singing something. All sorts of skin colors... darker and lighter. I am not sick... just old. I have no sadness. I lived a good life. It's time to go now."*

BC: *"What else do you see?"*

James: *"I am being picked up and floating. I hear a sound... something like a dog barking. There are so many entities here and all are very pleased to see me. I feel well. It's crazy how nice it is. They thank me and tell me that I have learnt to love unconditionally. I am happy."*

A few weeks after the regression, I had a phone call from James. I have to admit that I felt pleased to hear from him. He told me that he was about to board a plane that would take him to Perth, Australia. *"Just a holiday"*, he said. After our chat, James sent me a message. There was only one line *"Look what I am reading"*, followed by a photo of a past life regression book cover.

James and I still keep in touch and, to be very honest, I am pleased to hear about his accomplishments. Since the regression, James tapped even deeper into his own spirituality... and awesomeness!

CONNECTING TO THE LIFE FORCE

"Learn this from water: loud splashes the brook but the oceans depth are calm."

Buddha

After every past life regression, I give my clients printouts with detailed instructions on how to meditate. These days, meditation is a tool for coping with life in general because sometimes life can be hectic, as we all know. On top of that, as said earlier, meditation and hypnosis both focus on the theta brain waves' activity, which may help with recalling long lost memories.

Some of my clients enroll for further meditation workshops just because they want to make sure that they are doing it correctly; others become part of my advanced meditation groups that I run periodically. I enjoy teaching techniques to relax, and who would be better to attend than my clients who have already experienced past life regression?

So, what exactly is meditation? I am sure that you have heard the saying *"Praying is you talking to God whilst meditation is God talking to you"*. Meditation is exactly that; being aware of the present moment whilst listening to the silence around you. You may think that silence says nothing, but you are wrong. Silence is a tool of communication and represents an answer to most questions. The most plausible analogy that comes to mind is a conversation between you and your lover. Just imagine asking him or her if they love you, and all you get is a long moment of silence. You already have a clear answer.

The whole Internet is packed with meditation techniques and recordings that claim to teach you how to achieve a higher level of relaxation; therefore, some people believe that they can master meditation by just listening to the recordings... and for some this can be sufficient. However, before choosing a certain technique, you have to understand that there are two ways of meditating: one is called relaxation meditation and the other one, mindfulness meditation.

Relaxation meditation is something you can do by

yourself without any external help. I would even call this self-hypnosis. This is what I advise my clients to do in order to cope with life in general, and to make things easier for them I organized detailed instructions, which they all receive after a regression session.

Mindfulness meditation is a guided technique. In other words, there is a hypnotherapist or perhaps a meditation practitioner present, who runs the whole process. This is where the recordings on the Internet may be helpful. Whatever technique works for you is fine as long as you free your mind and block out everything that could create stress... and again, listen to the silence around you. It has so much to say!

My clients often ask how they can connect their inner selves with the universal life force. Well, this is a whole new story! In my meditation workshops, I like bringing people's attention to their energetic system - or chakra system - and especially to the advanced chakras. It helps them understand how the universal connection, or the association with a higher energy, is established.

I am sure that you have all heard about the wheels of energy called chakras. Just imagine that, as we have a circulatory system and a lymphatic system, we have an energetic system too. You may call this vital energy prana or chi or a product of ATP (adeno triphosphate). Chakras are the knots formed by the crossings of energy vessels - referred to as nadis – and are the central concept of the flow of energy through the human body. Therefore, I personally refer to chakras as our "energy organs".

I won't go into detailed explanations about the chakra system, but I will say that the first mention of the life energy was made in the Upanishads, which are ancient Sanskrit texts contained in the Vedas. The Upanishads mentioned two spiritual forces: *"Brahman"*, your own self, and *"Altman"*, the life force. We can connect to the life force or universal energy (Altman) through meditation. In other words, in our daily meditation, we can tap into the higher universal consciousness. Just picture your major internal body chakras as being your inner world, or your mind and body, and the advanced chakra, which are situated outside of your body, as being your connection to the outer world, or your soul.

You may think that your internal and external energy systems have nothing to do with the connection you establish in meditation; but they do. The seven internal major chakras are each related or connected to the seven layers of our aura, which form our subtle body. This is how we perceive the world around us, based on our own representational systems and how we send out messages through modalities of expressing ourselves. I am sure that you have met people you instantly felt that you liked or disliked, before even having any evidence of their character. This usually happens at the subtle body or aura level, where intentions are perceived and connectivity between humans is already established prior to proper contact. Let's just say that your auras integrated with theirs and you energetically or intuitively received a message.

There are seven main chakras, all based on a vertical line in our body, each related to one of the layers of our subtle body: Root chakra (Muladhara), Sacral chakra (Svadhishthana), Solar Plexus chakra (Manipura), Heart chakra (Anahata), Throat chakra (Vishuddha), Third Eye chakra (Ajna) and Crown chakra (Sahasrara). For our overview of the meditation subject, I won't detail the function of the major chakras. However, I will say that, during the years of studying the energetic system, I focused on the main characteristics and roles of these seven major chakras in what we call the internal energetic balance or, in other words, our inner self.

In traditional hypnotherapy, we work with suggestions and affirmations: we mostly use suggestibility tests in order to determine the client's receptivity to hypnosis, whilst we rely on affirmations for a positive outcome of the whole therapy session. Suggestions and affirmations work in the same way in meditation. Therefore I designed an affirmation that comprises all the functions of each major chakra in the human body. I usually suggest that my clients use it in their daily meditation in order to enhance the proper flow of energy inside their bodies. This affirmation is *"I exist, I feel, I think, I love, I express, I see beyond and I am one with all that it is"*. I truly believe that our own inner self, body and mind, or inner universe can be defined in this simple affirmation that refers to our human existence. It also gives assurance that we are able to see beyond that which our eyes can see, and remember our past lives. We are also one with the whole universe, defined as *"all that it is"*.

If the major chakras are in charge of our inner energy, the advanced chakras make the energetic connection with our outer worlds possible. The advanced chakras are situated outside of the human body and are important in accessing fourth, fifth and even sixth dimensions, beyond our human sight and hearing. These are the wheels of energy we rely on in our conversation with the outer worlds and are used in the aim of meditating. These advanced chakras are: the Soul chakra, the Spirit chakra, The Earth chakra, the Universal chakra and the Divine Gateway chakra. I won't tap into a detailed explanation of any of the advanced wheels of energy, but I will just mention that I designed an affirmation for my clients, based on the role of each advanced chakra, forming our so called *"outer world"*. This affirmation is *"I connect, I am eternal, I align, I can be beyond, and I am all that it is"*. I believe that this comprises our ability to connect and actually relates more to our soul's nature rather than to our human body; therefore, it represents being one with everything outside of that which our senses cannot grasp.

For my clients, these two affirmations define us as reincarnated spirits in human bodies belonging to our eternal souls. We are one with the universe and the universe is one with us. We are all the same and all connected at the soul level. We are eternal at the soul level! For some, this may mean that we are one with God and God is one with us. For me though it defines that, at the soul level, we are able to connect with the universal consciousness.

WE MET IN A PAST LIFE

"Love is composed of a single soul inhabiting two bodies."

Aristotle

I believe that our souls agreed to integrate or play a role in each of our lifetimes prior to reincarnating. That doesn't mean that we have a common destiny; it just indicates that we may have common paths for a while or that we are present in each other lives for the time being. I also believe that the reason this happens is related to evolvement and enlightenment. Remember that we all have lessons to learn and to teach and that this process cannot exist in the absence of a social environment.

First of all, as I have already said, the soul decides to be born into a certain family. Perhaps that family serves in learning the particular lesson we are here for. I remember a client of mine asking why his soul would have decided to be born into a family that treated him badly and abused him. What if, in order to learn your life path lesson, the only options were to be born into that abusive family or to be born without legs and arms? What would you have chosen? I am sure that things don't work exactly this way, when the soul makes the decision in the life between lives, but this may be a good analogy without excusing the abuse a family may have put you through.

I also believe that, as it chooses a family to be born into, the soul decides which other souls could play a positive role in achieving its karmic lesson. Another client of mine was skeptical about this process too. He asked why would his soul have signed a contract to coexist with a wife who left him for his brother. I am sure that souls look at the complete picture, instead of positive versus negative experiences in a lifetime. The whole process is to evolve and attain enlightenment.

Because of these unwritten contracts between souls, many of us may meet all over again in more lives. No matter how long we stay in each other's lives or the feelings we bring with us, the main thing is that we help each other learn what we are here for. Many of my clients recognize in other lives people they know in their current life. One of them is Nicole.

Nicole is a dear friend of mine. Ten years younger than I am, she is a tall, statuesque, beautiful and extremely joyful woman. She owns the unique art of making people smile. But that is not all. Nicole is also a very talented lady. She is a painter who dreams of being recognized worldwide, and I am positive that she will be, because she is a very gifted and determined woman, who knows how to market herself. There is something special about her; a mixture of mystery, softness, excellent communication skills and extreme joy. I am lucky having her as a friend!

Nicole is married to a lovely guy and together they are a formidable team. They may have had their ups and downs but have stayed committed to each other and have continued to do so.

Everything seems to work perfectly for Nicole; great house, loving husband, high level of spirituality, indeed an unreal talent... she has everything one could desire. This is no coincidence, for I believe it is Nicole's consciousness that attracts her abundance.

Nicole had a few past life regression sessions with me because she desired to understand her soul's journey through her past lives, and one of them caught my attention.

Nicole: *"I wear a uniform. I think that it is an army outfit.... different though."*

BC: *"Different?"*

Nicole: *"It's not something I've seen before. Even my boots are different."*

BC: *"What year is it?"*

Nicole: *"It's 1675. I speak a language I don't understand... Spanish, I guess. I am a man.... quite young."*

BC: *"Where are you?"*

Nicole: *"It should be a war, but there is no shooting. I am behind the lines. I am not afraid because I am not in the front line."*

BC: *"Are there any people with you?"*

Nicole: *"Lots. Everybody does something. Everybody is busy. I am organizing something too, but I am not sure what."*

BC: *"Is there anybody you recognize?"*

Nicole: *"Hmmmm... yes, my husband Dan is here. I call him Luis though. This is his name. He is a lieutenant. He is my best friend. We have known each other since we were very young."*

Dan is Nicole's husband in the present life.

BC: *"Do you have any family?"*

Nicole: *"My parents may be still alive. I haven't seen them in quite a while. I am not married, but Luis is. He has a little boy, maybe 4 years old."*

BC: *"So tell me what's happening."*

Nicole: *"Luis and I are talking. We share everything. I wish this war would end and we could have our lives back."*

I left Nicole for a few minutes to remember more about the war and I expected her to give me more details about the army routine in the 1600s in Spain. Instead she started panicking.

Nicole: *"Something is happening. There are some noises, strange noises. People run all over the place. There is some shooting. I don't understand how they got so far. We are behind enemy lines. They got to us and they are attacking us. I am searching for Luis."*

BC: *"Can you see him?"*

Nicole: *"No. I am searching. He is nowhere.... Oh, I see him now. He is down. He is hurt. I am running to him. It's him."*

Nicole started being anxious and tears began to form in the corners of her eyes.

Nicole: *"He is dead. There is nothing I can do. My*

friend is gone."

At this moment, she started crying quietly and looked so hopeless in the recliner chair.

BC: *"That's fine. You know it's fine. What is happening?"*

Nicole: *"I promised him that, if something happens to him, after the war I would go back in the village, marry his wife and raise his child. I promised…"*

I regressed Nicole to a moment later in that life. To be perfectly honest, I was curious if she kept her promise to her best friend.

Nicole: *"I am old now…. maybe even sick. Luis' child is here with me. He is a great son. It's only us here. My wife… his wife died young. She was a good woman and so grateful for everything. She was sick for long time and then she died. I kept my promise…. Luis was my best friend."*

A few minutes later, Nicole started her journey in the life between lives, a place of healing.

Nicole: *"I hear his voice."*

BC: *"Whose voice?"*

Nicole: *"It's his. He is here waiting for me. I don't see him, but I hear him. And there are many angels…. I feel so relaxed. I am home. Angels are talking to me. They say that I was honest and loyal and kept my promises. They are happy with how I lived."*

Whenever I listen to Nicole's past life regression tapes they confirm to me that she was and still is a very lucky person. She had found a lover who was part of her previous existence ... and perhaps of others too. They were best friends with life paths that have been inextricably linked.

In most cases, once a client realizes that a person who plays an important role in the present life was somebody close to them in a past life, the dynamic of the relationship changes. Many clients say that they don't take things for granted anymore. Is it possible for a soul to attract the same people in each life or is it just a matter of reincarnating in the same group? I am sure that nobody has the answer but the soul itself. However, what I understand is that we are born all over again in the same group of souls. Sometimes new souls, foreign to our previous incarnations, are attracted to or by our souls, to play a certain role in one of our existences. Maybe we hold the key to their evolution as much as they hold the key to ours; there is always a reason why our paths interact! I have seen proof of this when some of my clients recalled memories about people they already know in their present lives, whilst others talked about individuals they couldn't recognize. Again, souls recognize souls on a deep energetic level!

MARRIED IN MORE LIVES

"Love is the beauty of the soul"

Saint Augustine

Nicole was not the only client who remembered somebody very dear to her in a past incarnation. Lily's story is even more fascinating.

Lily is an accomplished woman. In her early 50s, she has a successful business that gives her a very comfortable lifestyle. Lily is married to a kind man; but this wasn't always the case. Her first marriage failed and left her as the sole provider for her two children. In the absence of a husband for her and a father for her children, Lily made the impossible possible, and gave her children access to the best education she could. Then, after a while of being single, she met a man who put a ring on her finger. Her second marriage was ideal and gave her peace of mind and healed her heart.

It was on a Friday afternoon when Lily had her past life regression session. I started talking while looking out of my practice window. The sun was slowly going down and the colors were incredible. The colors really complemented Lily's skin complexion and I focused all my attention on her. Once in a trance, Lily revisited one of her past lives and, when she started talking, her deep voice seemed excited.

Lily: *"I am in a village in France. I am a woman and I wear a very sophisticated dress. I am in my own home sewing something."*

BC: *"Who else lives in your house?"*

Lily: *"I am married to a man who has an accent, British accent. His name is Charles. We have two boys. They are just young."*

BC: *"Do you recognize your husband or children as people in your current life?"*

Lily: *"For sure. Charles is my husband John. He doesn't look like him, but I am absolutely sure it's him... same energy!"*

John is Lily's second husband in the present life.

BC: *"What is your name?"*

Lily: *"Marie. I am French and very beautiful. I am 27 years old."*

BC: *"What else do you remember about yourself?"*

Lily: *"We make dresses. My husband designs and sews them and I model them. But I help him sewing when he is busy. We live in a big house with many rooms. It's the biggest house in the village. We have many clients and make good money."*

BC: *"Do you remember the year?"*

Lily: *"Sure. It's October 1854. I know that for sure because Charles' birthday is very soon."*

BC: *"Do you remember how long you've been married?"*

Lily: *"I met Charles six or seven years ago; I don't remember exactly when. We met in Paris. We married in the village chapel maybe four years ago. Our two sons came one after another. They are young. We all live in this house that belonged to my parents. They died a long time ago, but I don't remember very well what happened."*

BC: *"So you are making dresses...."*

Lily: *"Yes. Charles is so talented. I just help him and I model the dresses. We have many clients. We are well off."*

I suggested Lily moves further down in time. She picked a scene that was relevant for her.

Lily: *"It's later in the day, almost evening. I am in the kitchen boiling a tea for Charles. I see the neighbors walking on the street. Our house is on the main street. There is an established apple tree in front of the kitchen window. It's blossoming."*

BC: *"Where is your family?"*

Lily: *"Charles is in bed. He is very sick and coughs.... something wrong with his lungs. He is not old... perhaps 69. I don't think he will make it. He is very sick."*

BC: *"Where are your children?"*

Lily: *"They live in Paris with their wives and children. We have three grandchildren, two boys and a girl."*

I moved Lily again to another significant moment in that lifetime, hoping that she would remember more about her life as a dressmaker in France in the 1840s.

Lily: *"I am in my bedroom and I think that I am sick or just old. One of my sons is here with me. The doctor came earlier. My head is very sore."*

BC: *"Where is Charles?"*

Lily: *"He died ten years ago. He was a good husband and I loved him dearly. I have never worked since he died. I had enough money to live a good life. But now I am old and sick, and my head is so sore. I have difficulty breathing."*

A few minutes later, her soul left her body and Lily kept silent. Then she started talking again.

Lily: *"I am floating and there is so much light around me. I see something.... maybe bubbles of light... or something else. I am not sure. I hear voices. They tell me that I lived virtuously, and I was a good wife and a good mother. I learnt how important family is. The voices sound like Charles. He should be here. I am looking for him, but I cannot see him."*

After the session, Lily said she had always known that she was in a loving relationship in a previous life with the same man she is currently married to. She felt that she knew everything about him from the moment they first met. You may call this déjà vu, but for Lily it was more than that.

For me, Lily's story brings hope that one can live more than once being happily married to the same person. Perhaps we pick the same people all over again until we totally complete each other; or this may happen only randomly. Why and how, it's only up to the souls themselves to decide.

REGRESSING IN A GROUP

"As I have not worried to be born, I do not worry to die"
Federico Garcia Lorca

One of my clients suggested starting past life regression group workshops or classes. I was quite skeptical about this, mostly because I thought it would be difficult to bring ten or more people to the same level of hypnosis simultaneously. I was familiar with stage hypnosis. I have even tried this on small groups in the past. So I started thinking more and more about regressing a group into past lives. On a side note, after mentioning stage hypnosis, I feel obliged to clarify that for me this type of hypnosis is usually used for the purposes of entertainment only and should not be confused with practicing hypnosis.

Following my client's suggestion of group hypnosis, I started investing time into designing a suitable method. You see, I am not a stage hypnotist... I was therefore wondering if I needed to apply an authoritarian method, whereby the group is approached in a more direct or commanding way, or if I needed to adopt a more permissive method, which involves giving more responsibility to the clients in order to achieve a trance state. I was also debating whether I should use direct communication, giving clear messages to the group and expecting them to act upon my instruction, or to adopt an indirect approach, using more suggestions and metaphors. So I decided to go for a mixture!

I debated with myself over the benefits and drawbacks of conducting group hypnosis, in a desire to find the best way I could to lead a group into past life regression. I already knew for sure that I could accommodate a small group of perhaps twelve people and that I would have to make sure I explained in detail what they could expect. Now, when I look back, I realize that I used a mixture of techniques, perhaps not all purely academic, but at the end of the day, everything worked well.

So here I was in my living room waiting for my group of ten ladies to arrive. In my experience, women seem more interested in past life regressions. It was a cold winter evening. I lit a nice fire and I organized the space with ten therapy recliners, making sure that everybody would feel comfortable.

The ladies arrived, one after another and excitement was in the air. I established how each client thought they perceived their existence, in order to discover each person's way of learning and expressing themselves. I wasn't surprised to find that some were visual and others kinesthetic. None of these participants were audio though, which made things a little bit less complicated.

I explained that, because this was group hypnosis, at some stage of the session, I would ask questions, but I didn't expect answers. So when everybody was comfortable and ready, I started inducing a trance and suggested they travel back in time.

During the session, I recorded on a notepad my observations with regards to eye movement and the exact moment when some cried or smiled for instance. I looked for deep emotions and I wrote down everything that I thought would help me understand more about what the group was experiencing.

After the session, some ladies were bubbly and could not stop talking about their experiences, such as riding camels in the desert, climbing high mountains, fighting in a jungle or just living similar lives to their present ones. Others were more reserved. One of them in particular, Lydia, said nothing. She let everybody share their journeys into their past lives but made no attempt to impart her experience. So I finally turned to her and asked *"And you Lydia? Did you see or feel something? Anything whatsoever?"* Lydia looked into my eyes. She seemed sad and I thought to myself that she might have been disappointed with her experience.

Lydia: *"Oh yes. I've seen everything. I know what happened."*

Everybody turned to Lydia and asked questions. Lydia was in the center of attention and I felt that some ladies even envied her for the clarity of her memories.

Lydia: *"I was in Russia in 1724. It was night and very wet. I think that it rained for many days because there was water everywhere. I was on a street and saw the lights hanging on some tall poles. There were candles actually, some of them burnt off, others still lit. I was a man and I tried to remember my name, but all I knew was that it started with "A", maybe Alexander. I wore very old trousers and a coat and had no hat. It was very cold too and I saw myself walking on the street and looking into other houses through the windows. People talked in front of fires and there was a nice silence."*

BC: *"What were you looking for? Why were you in a street on a cold, wet evening?"*

Lydia: *"I had no home and I was looking for a place to sleep. I was dirty and very hungry. I lost everything I ever owned. I remember that I had a shop in partnership with somebody, but it was taken away from me. I was on the streets for more than a month and my health was failing. I was hungry and cold. I knew that it wasn't long until I'd die. I was so slim. I remember lying down on the street and trying to sleep. My stomach hurt badly, and I felt pressure in my head. I started crying and praying to God to take me away. I didn't understand why my business partner took away my life, but I knew that he was a greedy man. I died like a dog on the street with nobody close to me. I felt that I had lived for nothing. I would have expected to have at least one person with me when I passed on. Just before I died, I remembered that my family, wife and children, moved in with my business partner and hoped that they were happy, even if they betrayed me. The experience was so vivid, and I know that that man, Alexander, was me."*

Lydia's life as Alexander was so different to who she was in her current life. Lydia owns a gorgeous property on acres of land. She is a successful massage therapist and runs her own business. Lydia has been happily married for the last 30 years, to an honest man and together they have three adult children.

After the ladies left, I thought that this would be my only group past life regression. But I was wrong. The same group came back for more. So I decided to organize an evening every month for groups. I kept the number to a maximum of ten people and, in time, it became so popular that I had to hire a small hall and let twenty people attend at once. To be perfectly honest, I consider a regression in a group environment just a taster of what one can experience. My belief is that in a one on one session, there is more attention paid to the individual and more can be achieved, but again, for one who has never experienced a regression, a group session could be the first step.

DISTANCE PAST LIFE REGRESSION

"A state of the soul is either an emotion, a capacity or a
disposition virtue, therefore must be one of these three"

Aristotle

I have never performed distance hypnosis. I have always felt that one of my duties as a hypnotherapist is to notice and observe my clients while inducing hypnosis and that this could be achieved only by having them in front of me. I feared that in the absence of well-known signs, I wouldn't be in total control. It's not because I'm skeptical about the success of hypnosis audio recordings or apps that inundate the Internet. It's more to do with the way I was taught, and the importance of observing the client's body language whilst being in the same room as them. Visual signs prove to me the level of trance I have induced.

As a hypnotherapist, I know for instance that the slowing of the client's breath or the rate of rapid eye movement are signs of the trance level, thus I aim to observe every change in my client's body language. I also pay close attention to my client's feet. From the moment I meet a new client to the actual hypnosis stage, I focus mainly on their feet. You see, our feet tell a story, a very significant one. The feet tell me the client's level of confidence or anxiety as well as the level of trance they are experiencing. Therefore, if there is any critical factor or opposition that stops hypnosis, I see the signs and I know how to bypass the blockage.

You see, our brains usually think in patterns and, for the sake of past life regression therapy, clients reveal their unconditional thoughts once tapping into their emotions. Therefore, I've always felt it was vital to be in a position to read these unconditional responses. As a result of this, I had never performed a past life regression via Skype.... until I met Sue.

Sue is a friend of a friend who I had an online chat with a few months ago. I hadn't heard back from her, until one evening when she sent me an email asking for a past life regression session. The only thing was that Sue lives in

Sydney, Australia and I live in Inglewood, New Zealand. Initially, I thought that she may be travelling and having a holiday in my country. So I replied and asked for more details. Sue's email came back instantly. She said that she actually wanted a Skype session. I tried explaining that this is something I have never done before and wasn't sure if I was able to successfully deliver an effective session.

To my surprise, Sue's response came in the form of another email, which was the proof of her online payment for the session. I now felt obliged to do a Skype session and, to be honest, I was curious how successful this would be. We booked the session for a convenient time for us both, considering the time difference, and I asked Sue to provide some information so I could better understand her expectations for the session.

When the day came, just before I logged in, I tried remembering as much as I could about Sue. She was a gorgeous woman, with radiant skin and big brown eyes. Sue had an established business in the health and wellness field and was well known internationally. In her forties, she never married, nor had any children. I wasn't sure whether she had planned to be single or if it just happened that way. Did her busy lifestyle stop her from focusing on a family or was she unable to find the right person? Whatever her reasons may have been, the situation seemed to work very well for her.

Once we had established contact, we had a little chat and Sue told me that she was about to sign a big contract with an overseas supplier, which would take her business to a whole new level. However, she felt that something held her back and was stopping her from making the decision to sign. Sue said it wasn't the first time she had been indecisive about an important aspect of her life and that anytime this had happened in the past, she asked her friends to decide for her. She felt that she had no voice when asked to choose. Because of this, she thought that her inability to stand up and make firm decisions could be an issue carried from a past life.

Being an organized person, Sue set up the space for her session before logging in. On my screen, I noticed a sofa and, next to it, a little table with a microphone. Then she moved the laptop closer to the sofa for me to be able to observe her. I was wondering how the whole session would run and hoped the Internet would work properly. Then I started inducing her trance. A good half an hour later, I began asking questions whilst the weather outside deteriorated. I was quite concerned about the Internet connection.

BC: *"What do you see, hear or feel?"*

Sue: *"I see people working around me. They are cutting grass by hand. I am in a kind of paddock, somewhere outside."*

BC: *"Look at your feet. Are they smaller or bigger?"*

Sue: *"I see baby feet. I am a baby."*

BC: *"Now look at the people around you. Do you recognize anybody?"*

Sue: *"I don't think so. I know that my parents are out there, maybe working, but I don't see them."*

BC: *"What else do you see or hear?"*

Sue: *"People singing about hard times. It's summer and the sun is up. I don't know anything else because I am a baby."*

I felt that there was little more information she could add at this stage, so I progressed Sue forward in time, to a moment when she may have been an adult.

Sue: *"I am in a house, a really old, damp building. It's 1800, in a village in England. I believe that it is an old farm house."*

BC: *"Are you a man or a woman?"*

Sue: *"A very young girl, just a teenager. I may be 15 or 16. I wear an old long coat over a grey dress."*

BC: *"Are you alone or are there people near you?"*

Sue: *"There is an old lady... very old. I remember her name.... Meryl. She is short and fragile."*

BC: *"Do you remember your name?"*

Sue: *"My name is Martha."*

BC: *"What are you doing in the house?"*

Sue: *"I am not sure. I just opened the door to the kitchen and I've seen the old lady."*

BC: *"What is she doing there?"*

Sue: *"She is shuffling around... maybe cooking food. Not much food... there's poverty in this house."*

BC: *"Who is she to you?"*

Sue: *"I think that I work for her and she cooks food for me and others. As I look at her, she may be my grandmother in the present life."*

BC: *"Do you see any other people around?"*

Sue: *"There are many living in the same house, but I don't recognize their energies."*

BC: *"Who are they?"*

Sue: *"They are not family. My parents are not here. Maybe they have died or perhaps they work on another farm. I don't remember seeing them lately."*

BC: *"Is the old lady still cooking?"*

Sue: *"She is baking bread now. She prepares the dinner for us. We work for her and she gives us food and a place to sleep in return. It's a time of poverty."*

I helped Sue move even further in time and she started talking again.

Sue: *"I am 22 now. I work on the land. It's a farm actually and we all do different jobs. There are ten workers, but we don't speak to each other. We just work."*

BC: *"Do you have a husband or a boyfriend?"*

Sue: *"No, I am on my own. I don't have time for family. I am very poor. I have only a dress and a coat. I don't make money. I just get food and a bed."*

BC: *"And the old lady is still there?"*

Sue: *"Yes, she is cooking again. It's dinnertime and we all gather together around the table and eat dinner, but we don't speak to each other. We are all very poor and tired."*

A few minutes later, Sue jumped to another time as Martha.

Sue: *"I am 40 now. I am burnt out. I work too hard and am very poor. I still live in that house and work at the farm. Meryl died and somebody else runs the farm, a man. He is harsh on us workers."*

BC: *"Are you still single?"*

Sue: *"Yes, it's better this way. I never had a man. I don't have time and I don't know anybody else other than the workers."*

Sue's life was hard and nothing exciting seemed to happen. I decided to help her remember the last moments in that lifetime as Martha.

Sue: *"I am 70, old and tired. I live in another house. It's very small and dark... just one room. I don't work on the farm anymore. I live in this house on my own. I think the farmer lets me live here."*

BC: *"So you are still in the same village."*

Sue: *"I am somewhere in Somerset. Small village...."*

BC: *"Tell me what happens."*

Sue: *"I feel very old. I have a small dog. I am not sure how the dog got here, but he sleeps at my feet. I am about to die with a dog next to me. Nobody else..."*

Sue looked sad and I felt for her. She had a lonely existence working so hard for a bowl of food and a place to sleep. As if a weight had been lifted, she raised her head, smiled and talked again.

Sue: *"There is so much light around me. It feels bright and safe. I am happy!"*

BC: *"Can you remember what your lesson in the lifetime as Martha was?"*

Sue: *"Not playing it safe. Move on and live life, I*

am told. I should have left the farm and done something with my life. Others left and ended up well. But I couldn't decide to go. Something stopped me. Find love and live life!"

After the session, we had a very long chat. Sue was sure that the lifetime she had just traveled to could hold the key to the problems she was experiencing in her present life. This made sense to her; she was very relieved and happy. I was even happier. It was my first Skype past life regression and I was overjoyed that the Internet worked fine despite the storm outside. I wasn't sure whether or not I would accept other Skype sessions, but one thing I knew for definite: Sue learnt quite a lot from her past life and she felt more confident, less anxious and more assertive.

I haven't heard back from Sue since the regression, but I followed with interest her accomplishments on social media. She is stronger than ever, and I just hope that she was able to make the right decision with regards to expanding her health business overseas.

And just as a conclusion… Sue was my first distance regression client. Others followed, and those times I was more confident with the whole process.

YOU MAY NOT HAVE BEEN A CELEBRITY

"Finding myself to exist in the world, I believe I shall, in some shape or other, always exist"

Benjamin Franklin

People don't really know what to expect from a past life regression. However, when asked who they thought they might have been in a previous existence, many of them hoped they were celebrities and surrounded by fame. They believed that wealth and popularity might have been part of each of their past lifetimes.

Before a regression, I usually ask my clients what they expect from the session. In most cases, expectations and reality are very far apart.

Some of my clients have admitted that they had dreamt of being Alexander the Great or Napoleon; others strongly believed that their obsession with a particular personality is because they must have been that certain celebrity in a previous life. You have no idea how many clients expected to have lived as Einstein, Marilyn Monroe or even Nefertiti. Not many thought that their previous lives were just average. But what is average really? Every human existence, as average as it may seem, is the essence of excellence.

I always wondered if it's ambition, determination and desire to be above ordinary that creates the self-illusion that our previous existences were mandatory in changing the world. What if it's only our own ego talking? It may be possible that our lack of sense and fear in the current life generates the dream of importance in a previous life. Ego is exactly that - a life based on not being able to find our own path in the present and the fear of never finding it: a separation of the lower self, mind and body, and the higher self, soul, creates in most cases ego.

I haven't encountered a client regressing into the life of a celebrity, actor, politician or artist. I have never regressed a client into Leonardo da Vinci's body! I don't deny the fact that one could have been Abraham Lincoln for instance, but I haven't come across that client yet. However, one of my clients who experienced a fascinating regression was Gina.

I have known Gina for a few years. She is another friend of a friend. In her mid 40s, Gina has a lovely personality. Mostly quiet and shy, there definitely is something charming about her. Gina dreamt of living close to the beach and, when the opportunity presented itself, she grabbed it. She called me right after moving into a beautiful house surrounded by acres of land with a private path to the beach. She booked a past life regression and was prepared to drive over three hours to see me.

Gina arrived for her appointment just after lunch on a sunny autumn day. I remember the golden light warming up my therapy room. We chatted for a few minutes and I asked all the questions I usually ask my clients. I mostly wanted to understand why she wanted to be regressed. Gina said that, since moving to her charming property, she had had reoccurring dreams. She also said that each dream was identical, and she thought that all her weird dreams might have been related to a past life. Then Gina started elaborating on her odd dreams. *"I dreamt that I was near a very large lake. I couldn't see where it ends. Then I bent over, I looked at my reflection in the water and I saw a face coming from behind me. I knew that it was a woman, I knew that it was from Egypt, also knew that it was*

Cleopatra, but I couldn't see her well enough to be sure. But I saw her mean eyes and I started freaking out. I was sure that she wanted to harm me. When I turned to her, the face disappeared, and I woke up". Gina said that she had the same dream for weeks in a row.

I explained to her that the life she may travel to may not be the life that encodes the weird dream, but she badly wanted the regression. This being said, I started inducing hypnosis. It took me a while to make sure that Gina was in a deep hypnotic state.

BC: *"What do you see, hear or sense?"*

Gina: *"I am somewhere outside. It's sunset, still very warm. I feel peaceful."*

BC: *"Can you sense whether you are a woman or a man?"*

Gina: *"Yes, I know for sure that I am a woman. I am 30 years old. I wear a heavy, long dress. The dress is light blue. I wear some sandals, very light and very different. I have long black hair, but I wear it up."*

BC: *"Look at the surroundings. What do you see?"*

Gina: *"There are no buildings, but I see some people. They look exactly like me."*

BC: *"Exactly like you?"*

Gina: *"They have dark skin like me. Not dark,*

dark.... just darker. But I have lighter eyes... maybe light hazel."

BC: *"Do you know who those people are?"*

Gina: *"No, I don't think so. They work something. They are workers."*

BC: *"Do you know where you are?"*

Gina: *"Yes, it's Egypt. The year is.... I don't remember, but I know that it is very, very long time ago.... ancient time!"*

BC: *"What are you doing outside?"*

Gina: *"Just relaxing. Nothing special. Admiring the sunset. I always do that."*

I instructed Gina to move further in time and started counting down.

Gina: *"I am older, but not very old. I wear a long dress... light color... like creamy color. I cannot breathe easily.... something is very wrong!"*

BC: *"Why is that?"*

Gina: *"I don't know. I am not too old, not ready to die and not sick either, but I think I may be dying."*

BC: *"That's fine. Who is near you?"*

Gina: *"There are some people... soldiers. They want to harm me, but I am not sure why. I haven't done anything wrong. I am on a cold floor. There is a woman just above me."*

BC: *"Who is that woman?"*

Gina: *"It's Cleopatra. I know her well."*

BC: *"Look at her and tell me how she looks."*

Gina: *"Not as you know her. She looks different. Her eyes are different. She is not very beautiful. She wears a beautiful dress though. She is watching with indifference."*

BC: *"You said you know her. Do you know her well?"*

Gina: *"I know her well. I may be related to her. I visit her often. I came to visit her today."*

BC: *"Tell me what else you see."*

Gina: *"I am in this big room...very big. I am on the floor and Cleopatra is looking at me from above. She turns to those people and tells them something. I think that she wants me dead. I used to trust her, but not anymore... she wants me dead. I think they poisoned me. I don't know how, but they poisoned me. She told them to do it."*

BC: *"What else happens?"*

Gina: *"I have difficulty breathing. They poisoned me. I think that I know something important, but I don't remember what. All I know is that I am dying."*

And she did. Then she started telling me about her

death.

Gina: *"I know for sure that I was poisoned. I see my body on the floor; Cleopatra is looking at my body. She doesn't care too much."*

Gina didn't look anxious observing her own lifeless body on the floor.

Gina: *"I now rest and I feel so good. I know that I trusted too much. I should have been more reserved, but I trusted too much."*

BC: *"So was trust your lesson to learn?"*

Gina: *"Trust was my lesson, but I trusted too much."*

BC: *"Doesn't matter. What else do you see, hear or feel?"*

Gina: *"I am taken care of. Angels heal me. I feel so good. It's so nice, light and warm here."*

After the regression, Gina and I spent some time talking. She admitted that she had the feeling that she was Cleopatra's mother. She also said that she vaguely remembered being the famous queen's mother, but that this was the first thing she became aware of after hypnosis. She was absolutely positive about that and nothing could have changed her mind.

I am not sure who Gina was in that particular

lifetime she revisited. Was she Cleopatra's mother or just a servant... or none of those? Nobody knows more that her soul. The soul holds the right answers. At the end of the day, it is of no importance if Gina was the Egyptian queen's mother or just an ordinary woman in her private suite. What is remarkable however is the fact that Gina found peace knowing that her unpleasant dreams were related to one of her past existences.

Is it possible that our dreams are fractured memories from past lives; and if they are, how, when and why are they released? Unfortunately, encoding dreams would be possible only in that very revolutionary moment when science has the right tools to define the concept of consciousness. Until then, anything is possible, and nothing is impossible!

FEARS AND PHOBIAS FROM THE PAST

"He who has overcome his fears will truly be free"

Aristotle

Some people live in fear. There is always something to worry about and there is always something to stop us from achieving our goals. There is a fear of everything and there is a fear of nothing whatsoever. The truth is that every thought and every action can trigger fear. We are just human.

Fear is a mechanism that prevents us from being hurt, because it is an emotional response to a threatening trigger. Let's just admit that fear is part of our everyday life. There is nothing wrong with fear itself as long as it doesn't transform into phobia. If you don't know what the difference between fear and phobia is, imagine this scenario. Picture that you lock your house at night because you know that somebody could break into your house. This is perfectly normal. But to go from this thought to getting obsessed with the idea of being burgled or attacked and checking every five minutes, day and night, whether the door is locked or not, is an unrealistic fear. In this instance we can talk about a phobia because it represents an irrational response based on no tangible evidence.

We are not born with any phobias; we learn them during our lives. This is why hypnotherapy in general is so beneficial for getting rid of phobias or helping *"unlearn"* them. A newborn baby is afraid of loud noises and of falling. These are the only fears we are born with; the rest are accumulated during our lives due to our own experiences and perception.

I have worked with many clients to help them release emotional triggers that have caused phobias. The therapy I use is part of the traditional hypnotherapy practice. But then I met Sandra, who insisted on booking a past life regression. She was positive that she would benefit more from this method of therapy.

Sandra rang at the beginning of this year. I met her a few days later and I was pleasantly surprised. Sandra was soft and feminine. In her early 30`s, she was a humble and compassionate woman. Blonde, with beautiful blue eyes, Sandra emanated an amazing energy. We talked for a while and, once she felt totally comfortable, I asked her to fill in a questionnaire that would help me understand more about her.

Sandra had an inexplicable fear of the ocean, which is quite unusual for a person living in a country surrounded by water, like New Zealand. Sandra said that she was a very good swimmer and that she had no problem with indoor pools, but when it came to the open water, an irrational fear took over her. She couldn't understand what stopped her from enjoying a swim in the ocean, but she was aware that, as years passed, her phobia was becoming more acute.

Sandra sat on the recliner and I started inducing a trance state. It wasn't long until I noticed that I could begin asking questions.

Sandra: *"My name is Lisa. I am 10 years old. I wear a dress and funny shorts underneath. The color of my dress is dusty pink. I wear laced up boots."*

BC: *"What else do you see?"*

Sandra: *"I have very white skin and long blonde hair."*

BC: *"Where are you?"*

Sandra: *"In a small town. I see the streets and ladies in long dresses walking. Just in front of me, there is a saloon."*

BC: *"So what are you doing in that town?"*

Sandra: *"I live here with my parents. I am an only child. I have a dog… it's my dog… just a fluffy little white dog. I am walking the dog and I am happy. I jump and run and the dog follows me."*

BC: *"Anything else?"*

Sandra: *"No, just walking the dog and looking at people."*

BC: *"Do you know what the year is?"*

Sandra: *"I've read it in a newspaper. It's 1907, somewhere in America."*

I progressed Sandra to another time in that existence and she started talking again with that soft, charming voice.

Sandra: *"I am older… 30 years old. I am in my house sewing something. My home is very nice; not too big, but adorable. I don't think that I have lots of money, but I have everything I need."*

BC: *"What do you remember about your family?"*

Sandra: *"I am now married. I don't see my husband, but I know that I am happy with him. Maybe he is out working. I have three children, two girls and a little boy. They all have blonde hair like me. I love them very much. They are out, somewhere with their father."*

BC: *"Anything else you remember?"*

Sandra: *"No, just sewing in my home."*

So, I instructed Sandra to move to another scene that may be relevant for that past existence as Lisa.

Sandra: *"I am 31 now. I am standing at the side of a lake. It's a beautiful summer day, very, very hot."*

BC: *"What are you doing there?"*

Sandra: *"Just resting beside the water. It's very hot, no shade. I feel so happy... I love summer. Maybe my birthday is in summer... yes, it's just before my birthday."*

BC: *"Tell me what happens."*

Sandra: *"It's very hot, the sun is right above me... very hot. The lake is calm. I approach the lake and the water is just to my waist. It's so refreshing. I step a little bit further and the water is just to my chest now. I still wear my white dress with some red pattern... maybe flowers. It's so refreshing. I step again and my foot gets stuck into something. Something is pulling me down.... I cannot escape.... just pulling me down. It's a kind of algae, I guess. I am underwater now and my eyes are open. I cannot breath. I am dying."*

I gave Sandra a few moments to experience her soul

leaving her body and returning to the place called home. She smiled.

Sandra: *"I see an angel in the light. The angel is calming me saying that I was a good mother and lived a good life. I've done everything as expected of me. The angel says that it doesn't matter how we die and we all deal with death as we can."*

She took a breath in, then exhaled and started talking again.

Sandra: *"I see trees... they look like trees I've seen before. They are very tall."*

BC: *"Look down at your feet. What are you wearing?"*

Sandra: *"I wear boots... slip on boots... and a kind of white shirt with funny sleeves."*

BC: *"Are you a woman or a man?"*

Sandra: *"Woman. My name is Anna."*

BC: *"How old are you?"*

Sandra: *"30 years old. I have very long, reddish hair, almost ginger color."*

BC: *"What else do you see?"*

Sandra: *"I am close to the trees. I am gathering plants. I have a basket and collect plants."*

BC: *"Why is that?"*

Sandra: *"I heal people. I do some sort of healing with plants."*

BC: *"Do you know where you are?"*

Sandra: *"It's north of England, early 1800s.... maybe 1801."*

BC: *"Do you recall having a family of any sort?"*

Sandra: *"No. I have no parents.... Maybe I am an orphan. I am not in a relationship."*

BC: *"Look at your basket. What plants are there?"*

Sandra: *"All sorts, but I cannot name them... plants and little flowers.... I need them to heal people. I make a drink out of them."*

Sandra moved to another scene in that lifetime as Anna.

Sandra: *"I am outside in a different place. There are people around me. They are judging me and accusing me of healing other people. They made a circle around me and are questioning me. They tell me that I am a witch. They are not harming me, but I know that they will."*

BC: *"Do you recognize any of those people?"*

Sandra: *"Many. They are people from this life."*

I knew that Sandra had meant that she recognized people present in her current life.

Sandra: *"They tied me up to a stick and they carry*

me as I am. I don't yell because I know that nobody would save me. I know that they will kill me. Wait! There is a man who is a friend in the present. He is accusing me too. They all say that I am a witch."

BC: *"What else is happening?"*

Sandra: *"They are carrying me to a big area of water. I cannot see very well… maybe an ocean or a lake. I think that they will throw me in the water. I am very scared. I don't want to die like this. They let me down now. I am not in the water. Oh, they make a fire around me and burn me. It's really hot and the flames burn my skin. It's horrible."*

Sandra started panicking and her skin changed color. A few minutes later she calmed down and talked again.

Sandra: *"Oh, there are so many angels here. I am not in pain anymore. The angels are thanking me for helping people heal. They are sorry for what people did to me, but tell me that I had to go through that. I know that I would do it again."*

Sandra's regression fascinated me. Especially talking to her a few months after the regression. She told me that she had been able to swim in the ocean. Was her phobia of deep water triggered in the past lives she recalled with such clarity? Again, her soul would know.

BLOCKAGES FROM THE PAST

"Life is a constant process of dying"

Arthur Schopenhauer

Clients tell me sometimes that they believe they deserve more from this life. Some argue that external factors have stopped them from achieving more; others say that it's their own fault for not striving for something better. Some clients even speak about luck and bad luck. However, when I ask them to define luck, they cannot. Perhaps luck is being in the right place at the right moment or perhaps this is not even the case. Maybe we are in charge of attracting or making our own luck. Jarrod was one of the clients who blamed his misfortune on bad luck.

I met Jarrod on a rainy winter's day. He came to my practice straight from work and was still wearing his work uniform. He was an employee of a company who installed power poles in the area. What I noticed first about him was that he was shy... and defensive. He tried many different ways of justifying his presence in a hypnosis practice.

After chatting for a few minutes, he admitted that he wanted to make improvements to his life: to study, get a better job, find a partner, and have children. He felt as though there was an aura of bad luck around him and that he might have carried it from a past life, because he strongly believed that nothing was his fault. A really nice guy in his early thirties, I thought to myself; if anyone can change their life after a regression, he can.... as long as he visits an existence with the conclusive evidence he needs!

Once in trance, Jarrod remembered a very happy life.

Jarrod: *"I see shelves of books.... many books. There is a small wooden desk and I see myself studying. There are books all around me. There is a window in front of the desk. It has been raining for days now. I know that because I spend many hours studying at this desk."*

BC: *"Look at your feet. What do you wear?"*

Jarrod: *"Some weird sandals. I have grey trousers and a coat. Very old style."*

BC: *"Do you remember your name?"*

Jarrod: *"I don't remember it, but I know that it's a*

short name.... maybe starting with B. Ben maybe?"

BC: *"Do you know how old you are?"*

Jarrod: *"I am 27 years old. I am Irish. I am a student. I studied for many years and I am very smart."*

BC: *"Do you know what you study?"*

Jarrod: *"History. I study History."*

BC: *"What year is it?"*

Jarrod: *"It's 1617."*

BC: *"Do you have any family?"*

Jarrod: *"My parents live very far away. I am courting a girl. Her name is Elizabeth. We don't live together. She is very beautiful."*

I asked Jarrod to move further in time and to recall memories from his life as the Irish Ben.

Jarrod: *"I am 60 now. I walk on a street and many people know me. I am a kind of mayor or somebody really high in this town. It's a beautiful day. I wear a nice coat and very fancy boots. I see a clock tower. It's 12:10pm."*

BC: *"Do you still see Elizabeth?"*

Jarrod: *"Yes, I married her. We have a daughter. She is 27 and married. She has brown hair."*

BC: *"Do you recognize your daughter as being somebody in the present life?"*

Jarrod: *"Yes, she is my mother. She even smells like my*

mother."

BC: *"Is it a good life?"*

Jarrod: *"Very good life. I studied hard and now I am a good leader. People look up to me. I married my only love and we have a good daughter. I live in a nice house and have a good, good life."*

Then, Jarrod recalled his last moments in that life as Ben.

Jarrod: *"I am in my bed. I am very old. Elizabeth is with me. She looks concerned. I am too old to live longer. She is holding my hand as I pass over."*

As his soul left that body, Jarrod started speaking again.

Jarrod: *"I am being helped by angels. I think they are angels. I feel fine, no pain. I hear a voice that tells me that I lived to my full potential. The voice says that life is about living, helping yourself and helping others."*

After the regression, Jarrod was melancholy. He kept silent for a few minutes and then he said that now he understood that he was the only one who could make changes in his life. *"There is no bad luck. It's me who's stopping myself. I can achieve more. I've done it in other lives"*, Jarrod said. He left deciding to follow his dreams.

I haven't seen Jarrod since his past life regression

session. I just hope that he found love, started his studies and changed jobs, as he had wanted to so badly, mostly because his regression in time proved to him that he could live the life he dreamed.

TRAPPED IN A PAST LIFE

"Not all what happens, happens because of fate. Something is in our hands"

Carneades

I met Tracey on a Sunday morning at a Medieval Festival. I am not very sure why I was attending, as I was never a fan of that feudal period in time. However, there I was watching people dueling, dressed in odd costumes. I believe that I was the only one wearing a 21st century dress.

I don't remember who started the conversation, but in less than a few minutes, Tracey and I were chatting about all sorts. She was enjoying the fair. I wasn't, but I liked her spontaneity. She told me that her partner was obsessed with the medieval age and that he was one of the main characters in the day's events.

A few weeks later, Tracey emailed and asked to book a past life regression appointment. She arrived right on time, dressed all in grey. She looked calm and I didn't notice any fear, anxiety or excitement. Usually new clients are nervous at their first appointment, mostly because they don't know what to expect.

Prior to the regression, Tracey told me that she lived on a rural property and that she dreamt of becoming self-sufficient. In the past, she had a full time job, whilst her partner was in charge of the vegetable garden, the cows, the chickens and the horses. A few weeks ago, things changed when Tracey's contract finished and she wasn't able to renew it. So her partner found a job and she took over managing the property. She said that she loved the freedom she had, but was concerned about money… mostly the lack of it. Then she said that she was confident that a past life regression would give her answers about her life. *"I've felt trapped my whole life"*, she said. She elaborated about her childhood and about how severe and harsh her parents had been. *"I felt trapped in my family. Later I felt trapped in a relationship with my ex-partner that didn't work and in a job I had never enjoyed"*, she said. She agreed that life had started being better lately, but she was afraid that something could happen that would trap her again.

Listening to Tracey, I just hoped that the regression would give her the answers she expected.

Once in trance, our hypnotic conversation started.

BC: *"What do you see, hear or sense?"*

Tracey: *"I am in a bush... New Zealand bush."*

BC: *"Do you know where this bush may be?"*

Tracey: *"Yes, it's the area I grew up. I recognize the bush."*

Tracey referred to the area she grew up in the present life.

BC: *"Look down at your feet. Are your feet darker, lighter, smaller or bigger?"*

Tracey: *"I am barefoot. My feet are browner. I am a young woman... just 18 years old."*

BC: *"So what are you doing in the bush?"*

Tracey: *"Nothing much. Just waiting."*

BC: *"What are you waiting for?"*

Tracey: *"For my chief... my master. I have to wait for him here."*

BC: *"Master? Who is your master?"*

Tracey: *"A man. He is a high caste chief. He is a trader. He trades people. I have to go with him on his trips."*

BC: *"What is your name?"*

Tracey: *"Moana."*

BC: *"So, you're 18. Can you see how you look?"*

Tracey: *"I have long brown hair... very straight long hair. I have brown eyes. I don't think that I am beautiful.... I am just me."*

BC: *"What are you wearing?"*

Tracey: *"Nothing much really. Almost nothing!"*

BC: *"I want you to move to another scene in the lifetime as Moana, as I count from five to one. 5...4...3...2...1. Where are you now?"*

Tracey: *"I see a gathering. There are fifty or maybe a hundred people here. I am on call."*

BC: *"On call?"*

Tracey: *"Yes, waiting for the chief. We have to go away."*

BC: *"Can you describe your chief?"*

Tracey: *"He has many tattoos and wears two feathers. He is fearless. Everybody is afraid of him. I don't remember his name, but I know that he has a family of his own. He doesn't take his family on trips. He takes me."*

BC: *"Do you recognize this man, your master, as being somebody you know in the present life?"*

Tracey: *"I think he is my father."*

BC: *"How does your chief treat you?"*

Tracey: *"Be beats me often. He tells me to behave and, if he believes I don't, he beats me badly."*

BC: *"Why does he have this power over you?"*

Tracey: *"I am a slave. He is my owner."*

BC: *"How old are you now?"*

Tracey: *"Early 20s. I am still young."*

BC: *"So let's move further in that life as Moana as I will count again from five to one and, when I reach one, I want you to find yourself in another scene in that existence. Where are you now?"*

Tracey: *"I am on a beach. It's somewhere on the West Coast. I am just standing."*

The West Coast of New Zealand is far away from the area Tracey mentioned before and I was wondering how she got there.

BC: *"Are you happy or sad?"*

Tracey: *"Sad. I feel trapped. I don't have a choice. I have to do what my master tells me to."*

BC: *"So you are on a beach. How have you got there?"*

Tracey: *"I ran away. I couldn't do it anymore."*

BC: *"Tell me what happens."*

Tracey: *"Somebody found me. There are some people with him, but I don't know who they are. They are taking me back. My chief is waiting for me…"*

BC: *"What else?"*

Tracey: *"He starts beating me. I fall and my head hits the ground."*

BC: *"Is it painful?"*

Tracey: *"I don't know. I am looking at my dead body now."*

BC: *"Just float slowly and let your soul go back home and find peace. Whenever you are ready, tell me what you notice."*

Tracey: *"Silence… twilight and colors coming all around me."*

After the regression, Tracey told me how sad her life as Moana was. She said that she recalled being sexually and emotionally abused and she knew that only death would have stopped the trauma she endured. Tracey believed that she carried that whole trauma in her present life and that, after the regression, she felt lighter.

I kept in touch with Tracey and noticed a change in her behavior. She looked, exactly as she said, lighter… and stronger. It is not up to me to say if Tracey's trauma and the sensation of being trapped came from her lifetime as Moana. One thing I can however affirm: Tracey felt better after her past life regression and more than likely fearless…

exactly as her master was!

TALENT INHERITED FROM PAST LIVES

"The luck of having talent is not enough; one must have a talent for luck"

Hector Berlioz

Many people confuse skill with talent and this is absolutely normal, as nobody can prove the origin of talent. So what is the difference between the two? Well, skills are accumulated during our lives; therefore we all have skills according to our upbringing and education. On the other hand, I define talent as an ability or potential to do certain activities better than others.

Most people believe that we are born with a special aptitude for something and that we may have inherited it from our parents or ancestors. I remember that many years ago, in Eastern Europe, there was a study done on this subject. The research – which, by the way, had no precise conclusion - focused on professional athletes, and it was based on the hypothesis that children conceived by elite athletes may revolutionize sports. I had a good laugh about this research with one of my best friends, because my friend was a former Olympic medalist, married to another Olympic medalist. They had two children who had no ability, desire or drive to be involved in any sports.

It is said that talent skips a generation. It may be true… or not. Nobody has said yet that talent might be carried from another life; mostly because there has been no research on the subject and even if there was, nobody would be able to prove it. I believe that, if it is possible to carry promises and contracts from previous lives, talent could also have started way before one was born in the current life. Tarah was one of the clients who opened me up to this possibility.

Tarah is a sophisticated woman. Both her analytical and creative brain areas may be very well developed because Tarah has a high and well paid position in a technical field and is also an extremely talented artist. For years she juggled her job and her art, and recently she thought that now was the time to focus mostly on her creative potential. But, as we all know, a thought doesn't necessarily initiate an action. Therefore, a few months passed and she was still dividing time between a demanding job and an artistic field she loved. She booked a past life regression, despite the fact that she had to drive over three hours to see me, just because she felt hopeless about making the decision to quit her job and dedicating her next years to art.

When she arrived, I thought to myself that Tarah was everything I expected her to be. She was sophisticated, beautiful, well put together and very intelligent. I liked her instantly and I enjoyed our conversation. She was easy to talk to and her voice was pure velvet.

I started to induce trance and hoped that the life she recalled would be according to her expectations.

Tarah: *"I see water…. miles of water. It's daytime and I am near the water."*

BC: *"Are you a woman or a man?"*

Tarah: *"I am a child… hmmm, a girl. I am about 12. I have black hair."*

BC: *"What are you wearing?"*

Tarah: *"I am barefoot and wear a cute dress with flowers on it."*

BC: *"What are you doing next to the water?"*

Tarah: *"I am alone. Just looking at the waves. It's a nice, calm day and the sky is so blue."*

BC: *"What else do you see?"*

Tarah: *"I see a house near the water. It is my home. It has two levels and it's beautiful."*

BC: *"Do you know where this house is?"*

Tarah: *"It is in France."*

BC: *"Are there any people around?"*

Tarah: *"I have siblings, but they are doing their things. My parents are working at the moment. My mom is working at the market and my father is a fisherman. They are very strict with us."*

BC: *"Do you remember your name?"*

Tarah: *"No I don't."*

When Tarah started talking again, she was already further in that past life.

Tarah: *"I am 15 now. I am in the garden. It is the most beautiful garden... There is a gardener next door."*

BC: *"Do you recognize him as somebody in your current life?"*

Tarah: *"Yes, he is my father."*

I knew that what Tarah meant was that the gardener was her father in the present life.

BC: *"What does he call you?"*

Tarah: *"He calls me Anne. This is my name."*

BC: *"What year is it?"*

Tarah: *"1840."*

I moved Tarah to another scene in that lifetime as Anne.

Tarah: *"I am 20. I am in a city in France. I wear a beautiful white dress and I carry a bag. I brought something to the city."*

BC: *"Is there anybody with you?"*

Tarah: *"Yes, my boyfriend Pierre. He is taking photos."*

Suddenly Tarah moved three years in time.

Tarah: *"I am in the countryside. Pierre is here. We are married, but we don't have any children. There are many people around us, most of them I know in the present. I am 23. I own a kind of arts store. It's a creative hub. There are all sorts of art items."*

BC: *"Do you remember where you live?"*

Tarah: *"In my childhood house. Maybe I inherited it. I love this house."*

BC: *"And the shop? Is it open?"*

Tarah: *"Yes, the shop is doing well. I don't think that I sell only my art. There are other artists' pieces there."*

I then helped Tarah revisit the death scene in the

lifetime as Anne.

Tarah: *"I am in a chair on my balcony. I am around 80."*

BC: *"Are you sick?"*

Tarah: *"No, just heartbroken. Pierre died in an accident long time ago. It's so hard to let go."*

Then her soul left her body and went into the life between lives, the special place where souls are supposed to return after each incarnation, which for Tarah was *"full of children's voices"*.

After the regression, Tarah said that everything she recalled made sense to her. She believed that the store Anne owned, full of art pieces created by her and other artists, proved to her that her talent might have come from far back in time. This may have been right or not, I thought to myself. However, for me, the life Tarah revisited seemed so much like her: calm and beautiful!

PAST LIFE HEALING

"World history is a court of judgment"

Georg Hegel

I am often asked what the purpose of past life regression is and how one could benefit from knowing what happened in another existence. You see, it's not about identifying if you were a man or a woman, a soldier or a nun, poor or rich, or if you lived on a different continent. These details are fascinating, but they don't constitute the essence of a past life regression.

The most important aspect is healing. As I've said before, some people go through a regression out of curiosity. However most people are unable to sort out issues or concerns in their current life, no matter how hard they try, and accept that there may be a residual energy they have carried into the present. They may be in toxic relationships they cannot escape from, have an inexplicable pain without any medical cause, they may feel powerless in finding love or committing to a relationship or perhaps they may be unable to hold on to their money, no matter how much they earn.

A past life regression focuses on healing. My clients are the ones who recall their memories and I am responsible for moving them to certain points in a previous existence, asking questions and recording our hypnotic conversation. I am just a guide, whilst they are in charge of how the session goes. At the end of the day, the client does the healing because the client focuses on memories that are significant or essential for their current life. My role is simply to ask questions which help the client to focus on details in their past journeys, including the moment when death occurred in a past life.

Usually I like to ask my clients, right after they have visited the scene of their death and noticed their soul leaving the body, where they were in relation to the body. Most clients, if not all of them, are able to see their lifeless bodies. So my next question is what are their thoughts about that particular life and what are their feelings about what they remembered. I would also want to know whether or not the people involved in that existence are present in their current life and if there are any contracts or promises made then, which have been carried into the present. Remember that the clients hold the answers; therefore, they know which aspects of the past have been carried on into the present and are still influencing them negatively.

Most of my clients go even further and sense evolved souls in the realm between lives. They remember or are told the lessons they had to learn in the life they revisited. If this is not healing, nothing is!

You may ask yourself what contracts or promises one can carry into the present life. Just imagine someone who had made a vow of chastity or poverty. The energy of a vow of chastity carried into the present may stop one finding love; the energy of a vow of poverty may be a blockage to having money. Just picture somebody, who after a fight with their mother tells her *"I will always hate you!"*. She or he may continue to hate their current mother or the soul who the mother was in the past life. Things seem complicated, but they are not. At the soul's level, everything is simple and crystal clear.

Again, past life regression focuses on healing and, in the absence of it, I am not very sure whether it makes any sense. No matter how many books about past lives a hypnotist reads, when we're talking about healing, every client is an individual; therefore, the therapy has to be based on the client's own needs. If they feel complete at the end of the session, and were able to break any bonds of energy that have been carried needlessly into the present, then the session was a success.

When I think of residual energies, I always remember Leah. I met Leah a long time ago and knew that she was a massage therapist. Despite the fact that she was skilled and practiced her job very well, Leah was unable to build up her business to the point that it offered her the lifestyle she wanted... actually any lifestyle. Leah was nice to her clients, very respectful, gave them a massage above their expectations, but none of them would come back for a second therapy session. So she started having doubts that massage was her true vocation.

When I first saw Leah, I noticed how "proper" she looked. She had short blonde hair, green eyes and a very nice figure. I don't remember her having an inch of fat on her body. After chatting a little bit, I noticed what a nice personality she had.

Leah was my last client one Friday and I was really looking forward to the session... and to my weekend. Once

I felt that she was in deep trance, I started asking the usual questions and Leah responded with a really soft voice.

Leah: *"I see a brick wall. It's getting late, but I can still see it. I am in front of that wall. I am just a little girl, 5 year old actually. I wear a little white dress. I am very afraid. That wall is horrifying."*

BC: *"Do you remember your name?"*

Leah: *"They call me Fiona."*

BC: *"Tell me about that wall."*

Leah: *"It's not the only one. There are brick walls around me and I am alone and afraid. I don't know what I do there."*

So, I moved Leah further in time and she started describing again what she saw.

Leah: *"I am now 14 years old. The brick walls are still there. Now I see clearly. I am in a prison. I was beaten a few times. I have been here since I was five. I have done nothing wrong. I think that I live in that prison because I don't have parents. I know that I have a sister and she is here too."*

BC: *"Are you sure that it is a prison?"*

Leah: *"No. I think that it is a place for orphans. I don't remember my parents. I know my sister and I know that there are other children."*

BC: *"What language do you speak?"*

Leah: *"I speak English, but I am not in England. There is a kind of weird English with an accent. I am in a colony somewhere."*

BC: *"Do you know the year?"*

Leah: *"Precisely. It's 1897."*

A few minutes later, Leah was even further in time into a scene she decided she wanted to revisit.

Leah: *"I am 17. Still surrounded by brick walls. I don't see the sun often. I am in my bed. I was sick for a while. It's morning and I want to wake up, but I cannot. I cannot wake up. I think that I am dead. I had to let go."*

Leah's soul left her body after a very sad existence. So I asked her about any residual energy, promises and contracts she may have made then, and carried into the present life.

Leah: *"I know that the only people I've seen my whole life were the ones who looked after us children. They used to beat me and I hated them. I asked God every evening to push people away from me because I hated people."*

Suddenly, I thought to myself that this may be the reason that Leah's clients never rebook for massage sessions. But Leah started talking again and I knew that she jumped into another lifetime.

Leah: *"I see horses…many horses. There are horses everywhere. I am on a field in England. I am 22, just a young woman. I wear boots, tight pants and a grey top with long sleeves. I have long, brown hair and a very pale skin."*

BC: *"What year it is?"*

Leah: *"1778."*

BC: *"Where do you live?"*

Leah: *"I live alone in a small stone building since my great grandfather, Sydney, died. He raised me. I don't know anybody else. The house is in the middle of nowhere. There is somebody who brings essentials to the area, but I don't know who he is. I am alone."*

BC: *"Tell me about the horses."*

Leah: *"I think they belonged to my great grandfather. I take care of them. This is how I make a living. I am always with the horses. I only know a few people, but rarely see them."*

I moved Leah further in time and she found herself in another scene in that lifetime.

Leah: *"I am 30 now…. still alone. I am riding a horse. It's tall and brown and very rebellious. Everything moves fast… then I fall. I think that the horse was throwing me off. This is the end. I am thinking what would happen to my horses, but then I know that I am not alive anymore."*

I went through the healing questions I usually ask my clients right after revisiting the death scene.

Leah: *"I lived alone. My lesson was independence and I accomplished what I was here for. But I didn't trust people very much and people didn't like me. I knew they didn't."*

After visiting two lifetimes, Leah and I had a long post-therapy talk. She agreed that the blockage to making her business profitable and having a secure clientele might have started in the existences she had just recalled. Her beautiful personality had sent out the wrong response to her clients, who had stopped rebooking. Was that an energy she brought with herself in the current life? I would gladly answer if I knew the right answer, but I don't. What I do know however is that Leah has now started having permanent clients, and her business has grown since her past life regression.

I keep in touch with Leah and see her at some occasional events in my area. She is still that respectable, soft woman, but I can feel her confidence growing at the same rate as her business does.... and that makes me happy.

DNA CARRIED FROM PAST LIVES

"Make the best use of what's in your power and take the rest as it happens"

Epictetus

Many of you may wonder if your DNA is passed on at the soul level, from one incarnation to another. This subject has got more attention recently, especially now that finding ancestors through your DNA has become very trendy. More and more people all around the world are getting their DNA tested with the desire to know what genealogy line they belong to. In the same way, those who believe in reincarnation may wonder whether or not their present DNA contains the genetic data of their previous reincarnations. To be honest, this is one of the most common questions my clients ask.

To answer, I would first define DNA as a carrier of our genetic information. This genetic code, which is unique for each individual, is stored mostly in the nucleus of our cells. So, as there are no two people who have the same fingerprint, no person other than you would have your DNA.

I believe that our genetic code is passed through generations by our ancestors in a very random way, rather than carried on from life to life. However, remember that we have lived all over the world in all sorts of scenarios, so who says that we couldn't have had an incarnation on our ancestors' genetic line? We may have been the tenth grandparent of our present self... or not. I am not very sure that I can argue whether this is or isn't possible. However, Charles thought he had the right answer.

Charles attended one of my workshops and approached me after the event. I thought that he had questions about the topic, but instead he just wanted to book a couple of traditional hypnotherapy sessions for his wife. So I started working with his wife and, just before her second session, Charles emailed me and asked to book a past life regression session for himself.

He arrived on time and told me that he was a former army employee and therefore was never late for any appointments. While he was completing the forms, I had a better look at him. Charles was very tall and well built and no wonder, as he ran boot camps for many years. Easy to talk to, Charles was loud and funny… personality plus! His reason for booking a session was quite ambiguous. Charles had no clue who his father was and said that his mother was very stubborn and wouldn't share details. He said that, as a child, he suffered with not having a male figure in his life, and later in life he realized that he might never find out the truth.

I was unsure that Charles would revisit a lifetime that would help him find peace with the whole situation, and I told him this, but Charles was stubborn…. even more stubborn than his mother!

Charles sat on the recliner and I started inducing hypnosis. Soon he shared memories with me.

Charles: *"I am a young man and my name is Daniel. I think that my friends call me Dan. I may be 25. I live in a kind of farmhouse and all around the house there are grapevines. Yes, the farm belonged to my parents. My dad died suddenly a few years ago and my mother passed away just a few days ago. I am in charge of everything and the property belongs to me now."*

BC: *"Where is this property? Can you remember?"*

Charles: *"It is in France. People speak French and I do too."*

BC: *"What about the year? Can you recall it?"*

Charles: *"Hmmm... 1715. Yes, it is exactly that. It's mid-September. I know that for sure because we just picked grapes."*

BC: *"Do you see anybody around?"*

Charles: *"I have three workers, but there are not here at the moment. I am about to get married to Anna. She is a very distant cousin and we have loved each other since we were children. Anna has a younger sister, maybe just 10 years old. Her parents died too, so we will raise her sister as our own child."*

BC: *"What is Anna's sister name?"*

Charles: *"Hmmmm... Charlotte I think."*

I moved Charles further in time and wondered if he married Anna.

Charles: *"I am 30 years old now. I am marred to Anna and we raise Charlotte. I am not very happy. Charlotte is pregnant. She is just 15 and I don't understand how this happened. Anna is destroyed. We don't know who the father is. All we know is that he is one of my workers. Wait! I see who he is. Oh no! It's my fourth or fifth grandfather. He is one of my workers."*

I knew that Charles meant that the worker was his ancestor in his present life.

BC: *"What does he look like?"*

Charles: *"He is the same age as me. He is turned with his back to me. He turns to me now. Oh, no. It's me now. He looks exactly as I look. I know now for sure that I am my own fourth or fifth grandfather."*

The regression continued and Charles recalled his death at an old age. He told me that Charlotte died giving birth and Anna and he raised her baby boy. Then we started talking about the weird memory about his ancestor being himself in another life. It may be possible, I thought then… and still believe that. Returning to the subject of our own genetic composition, I would just say that everything is possible and I am sure that nobody can prove the contrary!

THE TRUTH ABOUT DEATH

"As I have not worried to be born, I do not worry to die"

Federico Garcia Lorca

Many people I know are afraid of death, some even terrified of the final moments in this life, rather than what happens after leaving this world. For those who believe in an afterlife, things seem to be less frightening. For them, death just represents a crossroad between life and afterlife, and an endless hope of a heavenly existence.

Death is a natural process of life itself, and no matter how much we try to avoid it by keeping our bodies fit, our minds young and our souls happy, there is no way of denying it. We can choose not to bring life onto this planet, but have no choice in regards to leaving life behind. We were born and we will sooner or later die!

I usually ask my clients what their beliefs are with regards to death, and the most common answer I get is fear of the unknown. I have always wondered how we could be afraid of something we know nothing about. However, to be very honest, we should know what death is by now and how it feels to die because we've been through it many times; we have died, and we came back. The soul never dies; it just moves from one life to another!

What I find remarkable is that, once a client remembers how they died in a past life, the fear of passing over diminishes. This is the effect of re-experiencing death and realizing that it is just a normal process the human body is meant to go through. It may also be the reassurance that life never really ends.

In conducting regressions, I've observed that my clients have recalled certain experiences in a past life with a higher intensity than they experienced the death scene. They also remembered their soul leaving their body as a very pleasant and absolutely organic phenomenon.

For me, the most accurate version of the concept of death is through Hinduism. Hindus believe that the human body is made out of five main elements. Out of these, four elements (water, air, earth and fire) are released back into the Universe whilst the fifth, called ether, comes back or reincarnates with the soul and therefore continues in the afterlife. According to Hindu religion, ether or perhaps life energy, is part of our subtle body that contains our own aura.

We all wonder what happens after death, because nobody knows for sure what comes after life. For me, one thing is certain though. The soul returns to its own base to go through a healing process. If each life we have lived is totally different, the life between lives is always the same. It is a familiar place for the soul and it represents the real home for our souls.

If you were born in a culture similar to mine, you will definitely have heard the saying *"Nobody knows what happens after death because nobody died and came back to tell us"*. On the contrary, we have actually returned many times. Each time we started over fresh and tried to accomplish as much as possible. Then, we left everything behind and returned *"home"*.

I don't have a database of thousands of past life regressions as some of my fellow hypnotherapists have. They may have worked longer in this domain than I have. However, the subjects I have worked with had gone through all sorts of scenarios with regards to death. Some experienced a traumatic passing over by being buried alive, burnt, traumatized, whilst others died peacefully of old age. The only similarity between all these cases is at that very moment when their souls left their bodies. This is the moment when we, humans, release the energy back into the universe.

It is said that we all leave our lives and cross over alone. No matter how many people are around us at the second we die, we are the only ones who experience the release of our souls.

Perhaps sometimes the fear of dying is based on hopelessness. I remember one of my clients, a very nice elderly lady, who was totally dependent on her husband. They married fifty years ago and they have been together ever since. I believe that she leaned on her husband more than he did on her, but this was their way of having a successful companionship. Maybe because of her dependence on her man, she was afraid that she wouldn't be able to go through death without his assistance, even though she was well aware that he wouldn't be able to help her anyway.

We are all different as our individuality is based not just on our feelings, emotions, weaknesses or talents. Our individuality is also the product of the cultures we develop in and on the beliefs and rituals in our collectivity that constitute our upbringing. Maybe this is the reason why some people seem to care less about death, whilst for others this process becomes a motif of fear or even obsession.

No matter how our rapport with death is, one thing is clear to me. Not all of us may experience marriage, giving birth, being overly successful in a career or even being famous, but we all have to eventually face death.

IN BETWEEN LIVES

"What is freedom? It is a clear conscience"

Periander

I have never had a client who hasn't recalled at least one little detail from the energetic realm in between lives. Each of them revisited their death in a past life, felt their soul being set free and raised up to the place it belonged. Some called this spiritual space home, others life between lives.

I believe that in this spiritual realm, souls are healed after the human body has died. In the same place, in my opinion, souls decide whether or not they want to reincarnate and which lesson they are prepared to accept. I believe that we come back into another body knowing what we are meant to do and how to achieve it; but once in contact with humanity, we forget. This is the reason why we humans are in a continual search to find ourselves, and live according to the way we decided we wanted to.

The level between lives is fascinating and I don't think that there is one person who can define precisely how it works. I picture this space based on what my clients remember in past life regressions. All my clients so far have referred to it as being a calm, relaxing, silent place and all visualized a bright light. They all said that the light was warm and healing and they all remembered how safe they felt surrounded by that light.

Some clients described that they were in the presence of angels; others saw entities they weren't able to fully describe. Some heard music; others voices talking to them. Some saw masters; others spirits of people they knew from the life they revisited. Some heard proper words; others felt vibrations. No matter how they experienced the beings on the other side, all my clients agreed that they heard words of encouragement. None of them referred to being made responsible for not achieving the lesson they were meant to. This makes me imagine life between lives as a layer of love and tolerance, and that there is no hell.

My clients' experiences with regards to the soul's home make me think that the life between lives may represent the heaven or Nirvana some religions refer to. I believe that leaving a perfect place like this can be hard for the soul. Therefore, I also believe that our souls know that incarnating is not a one-way ticket. We are meant to return to our spiritual realm each time we leave the planet Earth and we are allowed to stay there as long as we need, before making the decision to reincarnate.

After visualizing the death scene, bringing my clients to the life between lives happens in a very natural way. Most of them are able to receive messages, passed from what they call *"entities"* or *"angels"*; others remember clearly the lessons they had to learn in the life they just revisited. However, my client Claire proved to me that things are not always straightforward.

Claire rang one day at lunchtime. I remember that I had just finished my lunch break and was ready for my next appointment. I decided to take the call and make it fast as I knew that my next client was waiting. Claire introduced herself and said that I was highly recommended by her kinesiology therapist, who she had been seeing for the last few years. She booked an appointment and, after I hung up I realized that I didn't know the person who had recommended me.

Claire arrived for her appointment early and was happy

to wait in her car. When I opened the door, I thought that she might be in her late sixties or early seventies. I also noticed how petite and fragile she looked.

We started chatting and she told me that she felt there was a sort of blockage in her life. She said that she couldn't explain why this may be the case because she had everything she ever wanted: a good husband she had been married to for a few decades, financial stability, good children and grandchildren. Being retired, all her efforts now went towards developing her spirituality, but she felt that she might be at a crossroads. Then she talked about a possible curse or bad karma, accumulated in a past life.

As I don't believe in curses, I felt the whole conversation slipping away, so I proposed to start the regression and began inducing a hypnotic state. While talking, I noticed how small Claire's body looked on top of the recliner. Half an hour later, Claire was ready to talk, without waiting for my questions.

Claire: *"I feel somebody very close to me. It is not a human being.... feels like an entity or a different being, but I have the feeling that it has a sort of feminine energy."*

As she was talking, I understood that Claire was recalling a memory from the space in between reincarnations.

BC: *"Can you see or hear this entity?"*

Claire: *"I just feel that she is here and I know this is because she came to check on me."*

BC: *"Check on you?"*

Claire: *"Yes. I feel that she wants to know if I understand what I am here for."*

BC: *"What else?"*

Claire: *"I feel my left arm very heavy and I know that the entity heals my arm.... Something must have happened to my arm when I was alive."*

BC: *"Is it uncomfortable?"*

Claire: *"Not anymore. There are two beings, maybe angels; I am not sure... they are still checking on my arm. As they do that, I start feeling my heart opening. I feel light and healed."*

BC: *"Do you see yourself, maybe your legs or arms?"*

Claire: *"No. I am a soul. I don't have a body. I left my body and am getting ready to reincarnate."*

BC: *"Tell me what happens."*

Claire: *"I cannot decide what's next. I have to make a decision.... I know that. I may just stay here for a while because I have to be healed and prepared."*

BC: *"Do you hear any noises?"*

Claire: *"No sounds. It's a perfect silence. The beings don't speak, but I understand what they want. They do everything that needs to be done and I feel so light and happy. We don't need to talk. We understand each other. My heart opens up even more to everything I have to do next. It feels divine."*

BC: *"Do you have any messages the beings pass to you?"*

Claire: *"Just evolve and be enlightened. Enlightenment is everything. You have to search for it."*

I understood that Claire's soul was not ready to decide if or when to incarnate; therefore it went through the natural process of being healed and preparing for the next journey.

After the session, Claire said that whilst experiencing what she called *"heaven"*, she realized that there was no curse involved in her life and that the only blockage she felt was simply a delay in finding her way in the search for consciousness. She said that a weight was lifted and then, more than ever, she was ready to experience whatever was yet to come.

Claire left my practice relieved and, after she had gone, I thought about what just happened. As I have said, all my clients usually revisit past lives first and only after that have slight memories from the life between lives. For Claire, though, the most important memory seemed to be from her soul's home. Things don't always work as expected, but they always bring the best outcome... even if we cannot see that!

Epilogue

HOW MUCH IS TOO MUCH

A regression into past lives is a fascinating experience. If you have had one, you were, no doubt, left with many questions about your purpose as a human being. If you have not yet, there is still time. However, the question most of my clients ask is how many past life regressions one should have in order to fully understand their soul's reason. First of all, let's clarify why you may want to be regressed.

There are moments in life when you may feel that nothing goes as required; perhaps there is a blockage that follows a certain pattern. You may even have reoccurring dreams or the sensation that daily events are déjà vu experiences. You may find yourself in dire straits and unable to find your path. This is the moment when you may decide that a past life regression is needed.

If during or after the regression you find out the cause of disturbing events or blockages, pains or fears, there is no need to go any further.... unless you really want to! To be perfectly honest, most of my clients come back for a second session and, with this second regression, they learn even more about their own life path. Some feel that they need to dig deeper and book another two or three sessions a year.

So, how many past life regressions does one need, you may ask. My answer is as many as you wish, as long as this doesn't become a habit and you don't rely on your past decisions to make present ones. Life deserves to be lived and you need to be in the line for happiness and joy.

As I have said, you are here to learn a lesson and teach others one. Therefore, you need to focus on your present life path rather than constantly going back into the past. Nobody can live solely in the past!

Your life is a miracle as it was in each of your past lives. You may have had a hard life, you may have been poor or ill, but still, in that particular life, you definitely had good moments. You may have been killed or had a traumatic death, but looking back on that lifetime, you also had your joyful moments. There were ups and downs... there still are. There were people who loved you and people who didn't.... there still are. There were people you loved and people you didn't... there still are. Life was a miracle then, as it is now!

ABOUT THE AUTHOR

Brigitte Calloway is a hypnotherapist, who lives and maintains a private practice in New Plymouth, New Zealand. She practices traditional Hypnotherapy as well as past life regression hypnosis. Brigitte Calloway conducts workshops and seminars in the subjects of Karma, the Law of Attraction, Chakras and Mindfulness Meditation.

For more information, visit www.holistichealing.co.nz

Printed in Great Britain
by Amazon

27318953R00126

The Subterranean Kingdom

A Survey of Man-made Structures Beneath the Earth

Nigel Pennick

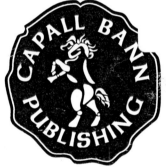

www.capallbann.co.uk

The Subterranean Kingdom

©2001 Nigel Pennick

ISBN 186163 073 5

Cover design by Paul Mason

Published by:

Capall Bann Publishing
Freshfields
Chieveley
Berks
RG20 8TF

Contents

Books by the same author, also published by Capall Bann:

Beginnings - Geomancy, Builder's Rites & Electional
 Astrology in the European Tradition
A Book of Beasts (with Helen Field)
Crossing the Borderlines - Guising, Masking & Ritual Animal
 Disguise in the European Tradition
Dragons of the West
Earth Harmony - Places of Power, Holiness & Healing
Lost Lands & Sunken Cities (2nd ed.)
Inner Mysteries of the Goths
The God Year (with Helen Field)
The Goddess Year (with Helen Field)
The New Celtic Oracle (with Nigel Jackson)
Ogham and Coelbren - Mystic Signs and Symbols of the Celtic
 Druids
Oracle of Geomancy
The Power Within - The Way of the Warrior and the Martial
 Arts in the European Tradition
Runic Astrology
Sacred Geometry
Secret Signs, Symbols and Sigils

Introduction

This book deals with man-made underground structures. By this is meant any tunnel, passage, denehole, shaft or crypt either hewn from the living rock, excavated partly below ground level and roofed over artificially, carved into a hillside, made in piled earth or bored deep through clay. I deal with all aspects of ancient underground structures and several of the more interesting and less well-known modern aspects, excluding on the whole tunnels made during the last two centuries solely for industrial or military use.

The value of underground structures has been recognized since the earliest times, when people found natural caves convenient dwelling-places. Although in Britain there are no great painted palaeolithic caves like those at Altamira or Lascaux, there is still a great deal of evidence of early human habitation. For many years archaeologists have excavated natural caves inhabited during the last Ice Ages and in Britain many fascinating finds have been made at Kent's Cavern, Torquay; Pin Hole, Cresswell Crags, Derbyshire, and Oldbury at Ightham in Kent. At Pin Hole, archaeologists uncovered a long unbroken sequence of habitation, while at Paviland Cave, Gower, they unearthed the remains of a young man buried with ornaments and the skull of an elephant (then a native animal), which had been painted red with ochre as part of the burial rites.

The remains of many now extinct animals abound in such caves, which are a rich source of information about life during an unimaginably distant past. Victoria Cave at Settle in Yorkshire and a cavern at Kirkdale have yielded bones and complete skeletons of hyaena, hippopotamus, elephant, lion, rhinoceros, bear and reindeer, indicating the deteriorating climate which preceded the last Ice Age.

Natural caves were inhabited at an archaic period in the past, but, as in all spheres of human endeavour, people began to improve on the natural. Caves were altered or extended for the convenience of their inhabitants. Not every cave is in the right place, and many places where subterranea might prove useful are unfortunately devoid of natural cavities. So it was that wholly artificial structures came to be made and continue to be made from the simplest cavities hacked into a cliffside to the most complex underground railway System.

Digging into the ground produces spoil as a by-product, and this may have an intrinsic value of its own. Mining originated when people digging at a mineral deposit outcropping at the surface continued to follow the valuable seam downwards into the earth. The realization that the earth could be exploited by mining led to a whole sophisticated technology of mining that has continued unabated to the present day. In early times, however, techniques were basic. At Grimes Graves, the earliest flint mines in Great Britain, shafts and tunnels were excavated through the chalk with nothing more than picks fashioned from the cast-off antlers of deer. The symbolism of antlers as emblematical of the male principle is well known, so it is perhaps appropriate that they should have been the first mining tools, penetrating the body of Mother Earth.

Such symbolism is obvious, and miners before the modern era of mechanization followed many rituals and superstitions in the course of their profession. Indeed, the knowledge of mining techniques was a highly prized skill, and the miner was held in great regard as a daredevil adventurer into the subterranean kingdom, braving the powers of the earth, both physical and non-material. Gnomes, Knockers, Yarthlings and other earth elementals were believed to inhabit mines, which were thus places of great spiritual danger as well as physical hazard. Even today unfortunate miners and tunnellers often lose their lives below ground, and in former times, safety was not held in as great regard as nowadays.

In addition to mines, underground rooms and tunnels have been made for many varying purposes: tombs, storage chambers, hypogea for worship and initiation, dwellings and passages. Many such subterranea are discovered each year. Most of them, unfortunately, are filled in as potential hazards before they can be investigated, so we have an incomplete knowledge of subterranea. Firstly, we find that some tunnels are purely legendary. Many of them are physically impossible, but nevertheless recall some geomantic feature of the district. Secondly, there are those tunnels which are only partly explored, having either collapsed or been filled in for part or all of their length. This type may or may not have associated legends, but will repay archaeological and antiquarian investigation. Thirdly, there are small structures such as underground rooms, crypts, cellars, vaults, chapels, chalk wells and deneholes. If these are known at all, they are usually well documented. Some longer passages and larger complexes are also known in their entirety or are currently being investigated, as at Nottingham. Fourthly, we have abandoned mines of various kinds, ranging from old coal workings to sand, chalk, flint, metal and stone mines. These have often taken on a new lease of life years after their abandonment. For example, in the two world wars, all types of subterranea were pressed into use as air-raid shelters or even underground factories. Several abandoned tube railways under London are notable for this. Additionally, World War II and its aftermath led to the construction of many purpose-built underground shelters and bunkers for both civilian and military use.

Everything mysterious has its own lore and legends, and sub-terranea are no exception. Across the whole of Britain we find the same stories repeated in different locations--the fiddler, drummer boy or piper who enters the perilous passage never to return; the animal put into one end of a tunnel which pops up, sometimes days later, several miles away; the ever-present wish for buried treasure; ghostly guardians of such hoards, and the sleeping armies of King Arthur awaiting the fateful day of resurrection.

It is probably no exaggeration to suggest that there are still many more undiscovered subterranea than those already known. Often, unsuspected tunnels appear with the subsidence of whole streets or housing estates, and sometimes such collapses are accompanied by tragedy. During 1961, a whole street in the Clamart district of Paris collapsed, killing twenty people. When the cause of the disaster was investigated, it was found that the roof of a hitherto unsuspected tunnel had disintegrated after a rainstorm. Paris is honeycombed with a vast network of these tunnels, some of which date from the Gaulish period. They are the abandoned workings of the mines from which much of the building stone of the city was quarried. During the eighteenth century a whole series of collapses led to the rediscovery of a network of abandoned tunnels under the Montparnasse district. These came in useful as a vast charnel house--a repository for the bones of departed Parisians removed from the overflowing cemeteries of the rapidly-growing city. The skeletal remains of over three million souls are said to be deposited in these tunnels, now known as the Catacombs.

Many interesting man-made subterranea have been discovered in various ancient cities during the construction of underground railways. Mines, tunnels and subterranean shrines as well as catacombs forgotten for centuries have been broken through as metro builders drove forward the running tunnels. In Paris, the construction of a line under the Buttes Chaumont disclosed a hundred-year-old gypsum mine with galleries extending 130 feet below the surface. The builders of

4

Rome's Metro have had to contend with a plethora of cellars, caves, catacombs, galleries and clandestine underground chapels, especially in the district between San Pietro in Vincolo and the Via Cavour. Construction of the second metro line in Rome ran no fewer than thirteen years behind schedule because of unmapped subterranea.

During the construction of the half-mile twin tunnels for the Tyne-Wear Metro under Gateshead, several old mine workings were encountered. Ancient underground 'roadways', which still bore the tracks left by sledges used to transport coal down to the river Tyne, were penetrated by the tunnel workers. Workmen on this section found relics of an earlier generation of tunnellers--clay pipes which were dated from their makers' marks to the period 1690-1730. None of the ancient workings had been mapped, and considerable exploratory work had to be undertaken before the construction of the metro could commence. Even deep-level tube railway construction is not free of such finds, for tunnellers under New York and London have broken into older, forgotten experimental tube railways dating from the middle of the 19th century.

The penetration of ancient archaeological sites, including tunnels, by metro builders was foreseen as early as 1902, when the Archaeological Society of Moscow protested against the proposed metro on the grounds that its tunnels would violate the consecrated ground of the ancient monasteries in that city. When the metro was finally begun during the reign of Stalin, to everybody's amazement a whole warren of tunnels, the semi-legendary Secret City of Ivan the Terrible, was discovered. As underground construction for rapid transit lines becomes more and more widespread, so many more fascinating underground structures will come to light. Recent discoveries of Aztec remains in Mexico City have shed new light on that civilization, thanks to the metro. Beneath the modern cities of the twentieth century we have a merging of the ancient and the modern aspects of subterranean construction, one stumbling upon the other to recall an earlier incarnation of the suterranean kingdom.

Chapter One

Tunnelling and Mining

Like most branches of human endeavour, subterranean construction has long been the preserve of experts. An intimate knowledge of the nature of rock, what can and what can not be done with it, is a prerequisite for burrowing through it, for to commence tunnelling operations without proper knowledge is to court disaster. Mining and tunnelling techniques have always been complex and not easily learnt, relying upon handed-down knowledge and expertise tempered by personal experience and intelligent trial and error. Although most tunnels are driven today by machines or with the use of explosives, such methods were not available before the last century. In soft rock, such as chalk or sandstone, tunnelling by means of hammer and chisel is not particularly difficult. Its only drawback is its slowness. In harder rocks, however, it is a painfully slow and arduous task, yet many ancient tunnels driven through the hardest rocks, such as granite, were bored with hand tools. For the hardest rocks, the miners in Ancient Egypt employed copper saws and reed drills supplied with emery dust abrasive and water. They also had tube drills which left a core of rock like modern high-speed drills. The most common ancient mining tool was a pick having one end pointed and the other end blunted like a hammer head. The pointed end was inserted in cracks, and the blunt end struck with a hammer. Wedges were also thrust into cracks and hammered, splitting the rock. A later development of this was known as 'plug and feathers' in which two plates of iron were inserted in a crevice and an iron wedge

7

hammered in between them. This method was popular in the lead mines in Derbyshire.

Although the Romans were the greatest ancient engineers, their tunnels were driven by the most basic methods. One way of dealing with hard rock was the costly and difficult procedure called fire setting. Invented by the Greeks, this involved lighting a fire at the working face, waiting until the rock was well heated, then throwing copious amounts of cold water or vinegar over the hot rock. This method of stone-breaking, used centuries later by 'Stonekiller' Robinson at Avebury to destroy the megaliths, causes the rock to crack and scale away from the surface. By such methods the ancient Roman engineers tunnelled through Monte Salvino. Other long tunnels, like that of Eupalinos at Samos, used nothing more than a hammer and chisel, but despite the primitive tools, the dimensions of such tunnels are remarkable. Eupalinos's tunnel is over 3000 feet in length and penetrates the solid limestone of a mountain over 900 feet in height. This astonishing early work also demonstrates the Planning techniques of ancient civil engineers.

Eupalinos began the Samos tunnel simultaneously at two headings, one on either side of the mountain, so that the miners would meet beneath the mid-point. His calculations were remarkably accurate: the two headings came very close to one another. Hearing the sound of hammering, the miners in one passage made a right-angled turn and then curved back to make the final breakthrough.

Documentary evidence of the survey work of the Roman tunnel engineers still survives. Survey instruments like the dioptra, the *groma* and the *libra aquaria* enabled the surveyors to lay out levels, lines and angles from which accurate scale drawings and plans were made. Sometimes the accurate work of the civil engineer was thwarted, however, by less competent contractors. A letter from Nonius Datus, the

Hydraulic Engineer of the Third Legion, to the magistrates at Saldae in Algeria, written in the year 152, records such an incident: 'I began by surveying and taking the levels of the mountain: I marked most carefully the axis of the tunnel across the ridge: I drew sections and plans of the whole work ...' But the contractors involved in constructing this Algerian tunnel failed to meet in the middle, as the designer was away on another job and could not supervise the work. Datus rectified the problem of divergent tunnels by making a tranverse tunnel to connect them, and the promised waters were supplied to Saldae.

Large scale tunnelling ceased in the west with the fall of Rome to the barbarians in the sixth century. Tunnelling and mining on a smaller scale then continued on a localized basis. In Persia and the Arab countries the building of subterranean aqueducts known as *qanats* has continued unbroken until the present. In the West also,techniques of well construction improved slowly over the years until they were finally rendered obselete during the 20th century by drilling.

Well-sinking, like all old crafts, had its own lore. After the appropriate site had been determined by a water diviner, a well sinker would be summoned to carry out the construction. But, as dowsers know, the patterns of water flow are affected by the phases of the moon, and no well-sinker of earlier days would begin his task during a waning moon when the water was in retreat. Usually the confined space in a well-shaft meant that only one man could actually work on it, which made the construction of wells a slow and laborious business. Every spadeful of earth or rock had to be iifted clear of the well, sometimes over a hundred feet, by bucket and rope. In deep wells, the accumulation of 'choke damp' or carbon dioxide gas was another potentially lethal hazard.

The construction of ordinary wells for drinking water is a difficult task requiring considerable skill. Near to the surface, the soil is usually of a loose nature which requires supporting to prevent its collapse into the well. In ancient times the shuttering was wooden, but since the middle ages it has usually been stone or brick. Such shuttering is known as *steining*, otherwise spelt steening or steyning, from the Old English *staenan*, stone. The depth to which steining was required depended upon the stability of the underlying strata, so once firm clay or rock was reached the steining was discontinued.

The technique of steining was ingenious. Before the middle of the last century, brick steining was constructed on a special iron-shod curb. This and the brickwork were gradually sunk into the well. Finally, the swelling of the ground prevented the steining from sinking further, and a new curb of smaller diameter was erected to continue the steining to the required depth.

Digging wells by hand was a specialist task, and extremely time consuming. When the well at Fort Regent in Jersey was built, it took sappers of the Royal Engineers 700 days between October 1806 and December 1808 to sink a well 235 feet in depth. They had to expend no less than 3000 Ib of gunpowder in the process, so even modern methods were scarcely more efficient. Nowadays, all wells are bored with modern drilling equipment, obviating the wasteful excavation of wide well-shafts.

The origins of mining are lost in the mists of antiquity. It is well known that primitive people at some time dwelt in natural caves, but there are also some enigmatic traces of tunnelling remaining from an archaic period of prehistory. North America has evidence of some of the earliest known mines. Their origins are unknown, but their antiquity is undoubted. In the February 1954 edition of the magazine *Coal Age*, there was a report of a discovery made during mining operations at the Lion coal mine in Wattis, Utah.

There the miners broke into pre-existing tunnel system which was so old that the coal residues remaining had already oxidized to the point where they were useless. In August 1953, John E. Wilson and Jesse D. Jennings of the University of Utah began an exploration of these ancient coal workings. The tunnels, they found, were on average five to six feet in height and followed the coal seams in exactly the manner of modern mines. In addition to the tunnels there were also storage rooms where coal had been stockpiled before transportation to the surface. One exceptionally large tunnel, eight feet in height, was traced to the astonishing depth of 8500 feet. No local native American tribe had ever known the use of coal, nor was there any tribal memory of it. The identity of the ancient miners remains a mystery to this day.

On Isle Royale, near the northern shore of Lake Superior, other ancient mines have been discovered. Here, the mining was not for coal but for copper ore. At Isle Royale, the excavations were again extensive, extending for almost two miles in a straight line. Some pits reached sixty feet beneath the ground to tap the veins of ore, and at one point the mine was worked through nine feet of solid rock to extract a vein of ore only eighteen inches in depth. Many of the tunnels were connected below ground, and drainage channels had been made to carry away excess water. Again, the miners are unknown. The mines, like many ancient artifacts in North America, remain puzzling relics of a forgotten era before the familiar 'Red Indians' took up a nomadic life.

The earliest mines in Europe are probably the oldest in the world. Copper smelting was carried on in the Balkans 6000 years ago, and remains of ancient mines for the extraction of ore still exist in Austria. In Britain, the flint mines at Grimes Graves were being exploited before 2000 B.C.E. The original form of these mines was a simple shallow pit, but later experience drove the miners to excavate a series of galleries from a central shaft, some of which were as much as forty feet deep. Flint was extracted from the chalk by means of picks and rakes made from the antlers of deer and shovels fashioned from the shoulder blades of cattle. Although the tools were later modernized, the technique of mining continued in the deneholes and chalk wells of southern England until well into the last century.

In ancient Egypt, mining was an essential part of the economy. By 1300 B.C.E. there were over a hundred gold mines in Nubia, the most famous being situated in the Wadi Hammamet. The deepest ancient Egyptian mine so far explored was 292 feet in depth and extended for a third of a mile along a vein of gold. Like so many other institutions of antiquity, mining was carried on with the use of slave labour. Diodorus Siculus, who visited Egypt in about 50 B.C.E., gave the following account:

"The Kings of Egypt collect condemned prisoners, prisoners of war and others who, beset by false accusations have been, in a fit of anger, cast into prison; these, sometimes alone, sometimes with their entire family, they send to the gold mines; partly to exact a just vengeance for crimes committed by the condemned, partly to secure a large revenue for themselves through their labour ... they are held constantly at work by day and all night long without any rest, and are kept from any chance of escape. For their guards are foreign soldiers, all of whom speak different languages, so that the slaves are unable by speech or friendly entreaty to corrupt those who watch them."

Such a bleak vision of authoritarian tyranny cast its shadow over mining operations for millennia. Even today, the semi-mythical salt mines of Russia conjure up images of hopeless wretches slaving to extract valuable minerals from dark and dangerous tunnels. In ancient Britain, the Romans opened up many lead mines, most of which were populated with slave labour. Most captive miners lived chained in subterranean

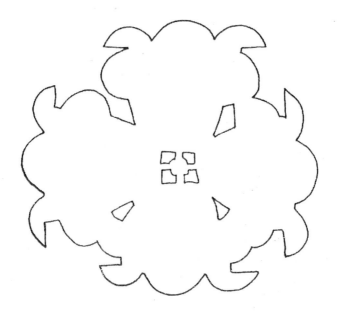

1. *Strange ground plans often evolved during specialised mining operations. This pattern was found in an 1879 flint mine at Brandon, Suffolk. (Nigel Pennick)*

darkness, and their life expectancy was short. It is little wonder then that concepts of the subterranean kingdom as a place of hellish torment emerged, for to be sent captive to work the mines was indeed condemnation to a life of unimaginable misery, a torment which ended only in death.

After the Roman period, mining continued in isolated parts of Europe. No major workings were contemplated until well after the millennium. Some of the Roman lead mines of Derbyshire may have continued in use during the Saxon and Danish periods, as it is recorded that in the ninth century the lead mines at Wirksworth were owned by Repton Abbey. After the Danish conquest, they passed from the Church to King Ceolwulf. The earliest accredited coal mining in Europe was at Zwickau in Saxony, where operations commenced some time during the tenth century. In England, however, there is no mention of coal mining in *The Domesday Book* -a meticulously accurate record of all resources in the newly-conquered realm of England - so it can safely be assumed that mining of this resource was unknown. Indeed, the use of coal at that time was not generally recognized. The bell-pits of south Staffordshire, sunk to exploit seams of ironstone, were made through seams of coal which was subsequently thrown back with rubbish used to fill in the pit when it was no longer usable. Similar workings have been found at Egton Moor, Yorkshire, and at Ponkey, Ruabon, South Wales.

During the thirteenth and fourteenth centuries there was a renaissance of underground activity in Britain. Techniques for the construction of deneholes were perfected, and coal mining took over from surface digging at points where coal seams broke ground. The first documentary evidence for coal mining in these isles comes from a charter to the monks of Newbottle Abbey near Preston in Lancashire. Dated 1210, the charter confers on the monks the right to mine coal.

By the end of the thirteenth century, coal mining was taking place in several localities. One of the earliest recorded mining fatalities was in 1291: a man was killed at Derby when a basket full of coal was accidentally dropped onto his head. The earliest means of obtaining coal or ironstone was by sinking beehive or bell-pits. These involved direct digging rather than mining, occupying a transitional point between opencast workings and true galleried mines. Bell-pits consisted of a shaft, generally about a yard in diameter, cut deep into the ground until it struck the seam to be mined. At that point, the shaft was 'belled out', being widened at the bottom to extract as much of the mineral as was consistent with safety. The limitations of the method was that the only means of removing the mineral was by means of a basket on a rope, either pulled up by hand or using a winch of the type commonly found at well-heads. No doubt the Derby fatality was in such a bell-pit. The basket which killed the miner would have been a *corf*, a circular basket made of hazel twigs. Corves were made with a wooden bow across the top which enabled them to be suspended by means of a hook on the end of the rope which hung down the shaft. They are illustrated in Georgius Agricola's famous treatise on mining *De Re Metallica*, published in 1556, and although the earliest documentary reference to the corf in England is in an order for the 'tithe coals' of Gateshead, dated 10 October 1539, corves were certainly in use many centuries earlier.

Although bell-pits were easy to dig and simple to operate, their productivity was low in relation to effort expended. Extension of bell-pit working was inevitable, and led to various aberrant forms of mine. Miners digging a seam of the Arley mine near Wigan came across such a pit during their work. It was composed of a series of polygonal chambers with vertical walls, each chamber opening into the next by means of a short passage. Although that system was unknown in Lancashire at the time and was thus of great antiquity, it was in common use in the thicker coals seams of south Staffordshire and was at one time employed in Monmouthshire.

The precise positioning of bell-pits is defined in the ancient laws of the independent miners of the Forest of Dean. The bounds of a man's mine were fixed as the distance to which a miner could throw the refuse from his pit - a distance later regularized as twelve yards all round. The laws, which date from about 1300 - the date ascribed to many Kentish deneholes--show that more sophisticated methods of mining had not then yet received general use.

Although mining in the Roman Empire had been a nationalized industry, mining during the Middle Ages was not

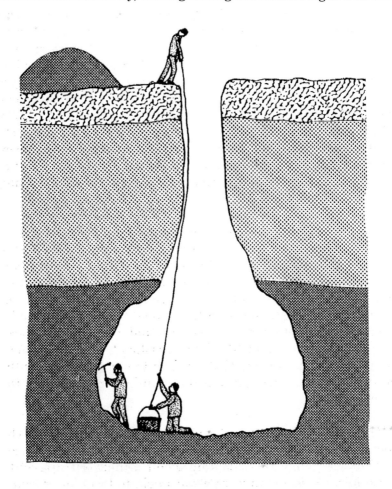

2. Method of working a bell-pit or denehole. (Nigel Pennick)

under government control. Although the monarch often had statutory rights to some of the proceeds of mining, the actual business was often restricted to a handful of free men. The dangerous and demanding nature of the work usually led to a degree of comradeship reminiscent of the *esprit de corps* and jealously guarded independence quite different from the slave status of antiquity. Metal miners in central Europe at places such as Freiburg, Joachimstal and Goslar were, like the Freemasons who built churches and cathedrals, exempt from taxation and military service. The tin miners of Cornwall and Devon and the lead miners of Derbyshire were possessed of the right to prospect anywhere except churchyards, highways, orchards and gardens. The Stannary Court of Cornwall had no jurisdiction above it - it was effectively a parliament. No tin miner could be compelled to plead beyond his own court, and no law was effective in Cornwall unless it had first been ratified by the Stannary. Today, many Cornishmen and women will not accept government regulations which remain unratified by the Stannary.

The lead miners of the Mendips, Alston Moor and Derbyshire also possessed their own autonomy and courts, but, by the eighteenth century the rise of capital shareholders meant that many once proud and independent miners were reduced to the status of employees and the modern era of labour had begun. However, in the Middle Ages the free status of miners made them at liberty to carry out contractual work in any place they were needed, and the characteristic of several unusual tunnels in Britain show that even as late as the eighteenth century the services of the independent miner were in demand.

Although the miners of metals were free men with considerable privileges, an unusual feature of mining practice is the difference in status between miners of different materials. Coal miners were always held to be of lower rank than metal miners, and in the seventeenth century Lord

17

Bacon and his followers recommended the use of felons as slave labourers in the mines. In Scotland, true serfdom existed in the coal mines until the latter years of the eighteenth century, only ceasing a few years before slavery was abolished in the whole British Empire. By this time, the peculiar privileges of the metal miners had been suppressed and all miners were of similar status, but it is odd to note that only the coal mines were nationalized by the British government in 1947, perpetuating the difference in status between the miners.

Chapter Two

Subterranea In Classical Antiquity

The engineering abilities of the ancients are well known. Their massive and long-lived structures still survive to awe the modern spectator. Such buildings as the pyramids, the great temples and aqueducts are continuing proof of the prowess of ancient engineers and architects. Among these impressive works are several tunnels and many other underground structures. Some are recorded in contemporary documents which afford an insight into the techniques employed by their builders, whilst some have been rediscovered during archaeological excavations.

An extremely early development of simple burial was the rock-cut tomb. It was in Egypt that this type of sepulchre was developed to its greatest extent, and the famous Valley of the Kings, where monarchs were buried, is riddled with many deep and elaborate shafts and tunnels. In *A History of Egypt,* published in 1909, James Breasted describes these tombs as 'Vast galleries, pierced into the mountain, passing from hall to hall, terminating many hundreds of feet from the entrance in a large chamber, where the body of the king is laid in a huge sarcophagus.' Huge quantities of material were excavated to create seemingly impenetrable tombs crammed with all possible requisites for the king in the afterlife. Such great spoil heaps at the entrance were magnets for the tomb robbers, and our one great complete tomb find, that of

Tutankhamen, was only intact because the tomb's entrance had been buried by the spoil from the tomb of a later pharoah.

A legendary but perfectly feasible tunnel of antiquity was that beneath the River Euphrates attributed to the Babylonian queen Semiramis. It is said to have connected her palace, which stood on one side of the river, with the Temple of Marduk on the opposite bank. Now although tunnelling directly beneath rivers was not feasible before the nineteenth century when Marc Brunel built the Thames Tunnel from Rotherhithe to Wapping (1825-43), this problem was circumvented in an ingenious manner. The Babylonian engineers diverted the wintertime trickle of the river into a specially constructed alternative channel before commencing the tunnel. A trench was made in the dry river bed, and a brick arch constructed in the manner of the time, sealed, and the river allowed to flow again in its old channel over the roof of the tunnel.

The Greek historian Diodorus Siculus puts the date of this tunnel at 2000 B.C., but the Semiramis known to history was an Assyrian queen of the eighth century B.C.E., so the facts are rather garbled. The techniques, however, were not beyond the civil engineers of the period, so there is probably a kernel of truth in the story. It was a common practice to connect religious sites to other buildings by secret passages, and several examples still survive in Britain.

In the eighth century B.C.E., the Israelite king Hezekiah, apprehensive of a possible siege of Jerusalem by the Assyrians, decided to safe- guard the city's water supply. The main spring at Gihon which provided Jerusalem's water was outside the city walls, so the king Ordered the construction of a tunnel from this source to the Pool of Siloam. The pool itself, formerly also outside the city wall, was then protected by new walls.

Hezekiah's tunnel ran in a wide curve from the well, beneath the walls of the city. Although it was only a few hundred feet in length, it was nevertheless a real achievement in engineering terms. Tunnelling began at each end. Miscalculations made the tunnels slightly out of alignment, but the miners, hearing the noise of each others' work, tunnelled towards one another and joined up. In 1880, an inscription in Phoenician characters recounting the construction was found on an inner wall of the tunnel. The use of Phoenician shows that Hezekiah, like Solomon before him, employed Phoenician expertise in his engineering works

A century after Hezekiah, another major subterranean aqueduct was built, this time by the Greeks. The historian Herodotus describes it as part of the water supply for the City of Samos. The tunnel was 'a double mouthed channel pierced... through the base of a high hill; the whole channel is seven furlongs in length, eight feet high and eight feet wide; and throughout the whole length there runs another channel twenty cubits deep and three feet wide through which the water coming from an abundant spring is carried by its pipes to the city of Samos. The designer of the work was Eupalinos, son of Naustrophos, a Megarian. For centuries, the tunnel was known only from documentary sources, but it was finally rediscovered in 1881.

Of all ancient civilizations, that of Rome is famed above all for its engineering prowess. The expertise of the *agrimensores,* the corps of geomantic surveyors who laid out newly-colonized territory, can be seen to this day. Part of the colonization process was the bringing of vast tracts of previously barren land under cultivation by the expedient of providing adequate water for irrigation. Throughout Italy, the Balkans and North Africa, the remains of Roman aqueducts can be found. The large and complex system which served the city of Rome still survives in fragments substantial enough to demonstrate the ability of its builders. Much of this system was constructed by

Sextus Julius Frontinus, perhaps the greatest of Roman civil engineers, some of whose writings still survive in the *Corpus Agrimensorum*, a compilation of Roman treatises on surveying and geomancy.

Like many hydraulic engineers, Frontinus was a professional soldier. In his military role, he rose to a high position and was appointed Governor of Britain in A.D. 80. When on his retirement from military service in A.D. 95 he was appointed *Curator Aquarum,* Chief Water Engineer of Rome, he immediately put new works in hand, being finally responsible for the construction of nine new aqueducts. Totalling 263 miles in length, these aqueducts were in the main either carried on arches or underground in tunnels. The Appian Aqueduct, for example, was subterranean for ten of its sixteen miles. Tunnelling was by this time a fine art which was not to be lost until the fall of the Empire several centuries later.

A major work constructed by Roman hydraulic engineers outside Italy was Hadrian's Aqueduct in Athens. No less than fifteen miles in length, this tunnel was a major feat of planning and execution. It was begun in about the year 115 and finished in the remarkably short time of six years, its miners sinking no fewer than 700 vertical shafts at intervals, their depths ranging from 30 to 130 feet. This enabled tunnelling to proceed on an heroic scale, the tunnel being pushed forward at scores of faces at the same time. Forgotten during the long decline under Turkish rule, Hadrian's Aqueduct was rediscovered in about 1840 and refurbished for further use. In 1925 it was again cleaned and repaired by Ulen and Company, an American firm of contractors, and today serves the city as a lasting tribute to ancient engineering.

Another major Roman tunnel was that driven through Monte Salvino. Pliny the Elder and Suetonius describe this work, an aqueduct built to carry water from Lake Fucinus (now called

Celano) to the River Liris (now Gangliano). From 22 shafts, some a massive 400 feet deep, a tunnel $3\frac{1}{2}$ miles in length was driven. Suetonius tells us that the construction, which was completed in the reign of the emperor Claudius, took the labour of 30,000 men for eleven years. During the Middle Ages, when the breakdown of organization led to the abandonment of so many ancient engineering masterpieces, the tunnel became blocked. It was re- opened during the last century when Prince Torlonia drained the lake.

Although the longest and most spectacular Roman tunnels were aqueducts, tunnelling for human access was also occasionally done. The resort of Baiae, seat of oracles and frequented by emperors and other Roman worthies, was difficult to get to because it was cut off from the city of Neapolis (Naples) by a rocky ridge. This Posilipan Ridge was such an awkward barrier that the emperor Augustus ordered an engineer named Cocceius to drive two tunnels through it - the Grotta de Seiano and the Grotta de Posilipo. Seneca and Petronius refer to the latter by its alternative names of Crypta Neapolitana, being the more unpleasant of the two and employed by the common folk whilst the Grotta de Seiano was reserved for the emperor and his entourage.

Both tunnels are about half a mile in length, but only the Grotta de Seiano was provided with shafts for illumination by sunlight. According to Seneca, the Posilipo was far less congenial. 'There is no prison longer than that *crypta,* no torch dimmer than those they shielded before us, which served not to lighten the darkness but only to look upon one another. In any case, if there had been a glimmer of light, the dust would have robbed us of it; it was dense enough to darken a place out of doors ...' So unpleasant were the conditions in ancient tunnels that they were used only where no other form of access would do.

Tunnelling was an integral part of ancient warfare, as mines were driven from places out of range of the enemy's weapons and extended to undermine the walls of besieged towns. Undermining involved literally mining beneath the walls, filling the space with combustible material and then setting it alight. As the tunnel collapsed, so did the walls. As early as 396 B.C.E. the last Etruscan town,Veii, was taken by sappers who tunnelled beneath the impregnable walls to admit the Roman besiegers.

The development of military mining was followed rapidly by the technique of counter-mining, as recorded by the Roman architectural writer Vitruvius, who tells of the siege of Marseilles in 49 B.C.E.:

When Marseilles was besieged and the enemy drove more than thirty tunnels, the inhabitants were on their guard, and made a deeper ditch than that in front of the rampart. But where inside the wall a ditch could not be made, they dug a moat, like a fish pond of great length and depth, over against the quarter where the tunnels were being dug, and filled it from the wells and harbour. Hence when a tunnel had its passages suddenly opened, a strong rush of water flooded in and threw down the pitprops. The troops inside were overwhelmed by the collapse of the tunnel and the flood of water.

Such mining and countermining was a feature of sieges well into the last century, and the modern 'mine' -an explosive charge buried in the ground - is a development of gunpowder in tunnels. Exercises in military mining were carried out at the Lines at Chatham, Kent, annually between the years 1816 and 1914, leaving a massive but unmapped system extending for many miles, but by 1914, sieges of that type were a thing of the past.

In addition to tombs, aqueducts, pedestrian tunnels and military mines, the tunnel engineers of ancient times also

24

excavated sacred places of worship and initiation. The Oracle of the Dead at Baiae and the Grotto of the Cumaean Sybil are two famous hypogea of antiquity, the latter, described by Virgil, having been excavated in the Monte de Cuma near Lake Avernus during the fifth or sixth century B.C. Oracles were almost invariably associated with subterranea, that at Delphi being above a cleft in the ground, the downward link to the infernal regions. Where such a natural cavern did not exist, the tunnellers made an artificial one whose plan coincided with the legendary geography of the underworld. In *The Aeneid,* Virgil writes:

Then Aeneas climbed the rocky hill
Where, on the crest the Temple of Apollo stands,
And there the fearsome cavern of the awesome Sybil lies,
Whence came her prophecies,
Inspired by great Delius himself.

In 1932, Amadeo Maiuri, following Virgil's account, excavated the fearsome cavern. He found it to be 450 feet in length, oriented true north-south with the *cella* of the Sybil at the southern end. When it was excavated, another Roman gallery 600 feet in length was found penetrating the Monte de Cuma at its base from east to west. This was part of a military road constructed by the master tunneller Cocceius and connected with a similar tunnel beneath Monte Grillo. The driving of a profane and functional tunnel through a holy mountain makes it likely that the grotto had been sealed by the time of Augustus.

The nearby Oracle of the Dead at Baiae certainly had been sealed by the time of Cocceius, the shrines of Apollo at Avernus and Baiae having been suppressed by the admiral Agrippa in about 35 B.C.E. during the Roman civil war. He decided that the religion of Apollo should be eradicated and in order to achieve its suppression he cut down the sacred groves on the shore of Lake Avernus. With the holy wood he built more ships for the navy, and Apollo's shrines were razed and replaced by naval dockyards. Such desecration appalled the god's devotees. The image of Apollo at Rome was seen to sweat and a massive storm occurred in the Bay of Naples. It raged for so long that the Pontifex Maximus was obliged to quell it by sacrificing a hecatomb of victims to the god.

Terrified by these manifestations, Agrippa temporarily halted the orgy of destruction, and instead of razing the rest of the shrine, he ordered that the vast subterranean passage system of the Oracle of the Dead should be filled in, and the surface shrine-rooms converted into hot baths. Thus the pilgrim town became a health resort. So that the Oracle's tunnels could never be used again, Agrippa's workmen packed them with a staggering 700 cubic yards of earth - 30 000 basketsful - for to merely brick up the entrance would have enabled it to be reopened at a later date. Thousands of man-hours spent in sealing the tunnels destroyed them for ever.

To attract such attention from its despoilers, the oracular tunnel system must have been of supreme importance. The shrine was in the form of a network of man-made passages corresponded with the legendary geography of the Realm of the Dead. It existed as early as the time of Homer, about 1000 B.C.E., and Strabo, writing a few years after its final suppression, refers to that writer: 'The people prior to my time were wont to make Avernus the setting of the fabulous story of *The Odyssey*; and moreover writers tell us that there was actually an oracle of the dead there, and that Odysseus visited it.' The oracle was attended by troglodyte priests who 'live on what they can get from mining, and from those who consult the oracle, which is situated far beneath the earth. And those who live about the oracle have a traditional custom that no one should see the sun but should only go outside the caverns at night.'

The entry to this microcosmic underworld was at the north-west corner of the Temple of Apollo, a quadrant of the cosmos which was geomantically dedicated to the Fates and the denizens of the underworld. The inner sanctuary is oriented towards midsummer sunset, symbolic of the annual death of nature. From the entrance to the inner *sanctum* the tunnel was 600 feet long, so that entering it must have been an awesome and terrifying ordeal. The power of such places was so great that they could never die naturally; those who wished to stop their use were forced to take drastic measures. We will meet similar cases in later chapters.

Chapter Three

The Religious Uses of Subterranea

Underground structures are ideal for the observance of religious rites. They provide mysterious and secret places in which to carry out initiations and rituals requiring long and unbroken periods of observance hidden from the prying eyes of the profane. All the legends of the underworld equate this subterranean kingdom with the realm of death from which most never return. This is a natural consequence of the practice of the burial of the dead which has been a human custom for hundreds of thousand of years. The earliest subterranean structures of religious use may have been tombs where services were held for the departed, but many chambered cairns and long barrows in northern Europe, whilst used for burial, also show unmistakable traces of serving the living in their worship.

It is a risky business to enter an underground place, where all kinds of unforseen hazards may lurk. The legends of Orpheus and other penetrators of the subterranean kingdom were paralleled in the world of the living by the initiatory rites performed inside real subterranea, which included natural caves in which the numinous qualities of the earth could be felt. Such places were often the haunt of oracles, as in the Grotto of the Cumaean Sybil or the cave of Ramahavaly at Andringitra in Madagascar. It is certain that the descriptions of the underworld so confidently given by ancient authors are in fact expositions of the subterranean geography of initiatory and oracular hypogea.

Many legendary subterranea were linked with the upper as well as the lower world. They were often placed at the point where the three worlds - upper, middle and lower - were believed to have contact by way of the world axial tree, the central *omphalos* linking all time and space at one point. This contact existed in more than a symbolic or conceptual way. Underground structures may at first appear most unpromising places for the observation of the heavens, yet this was precisely their use in many places.

It has often been stated that the ancient Druids used to observe the passage of the heavens from the bottom of wells, hence the saying 'Truth lies at the bottom of a well'. The modern native American Hopi tribe still observes the stars through the vertical shafts of their *kivas* or underground shrine rooms. The interiors of the so-called 'passage graves' of Europe have long been held in local tradition to have been sites of religious observance in ancient times. Vast chambers, approached by long passages exist in many important barrows, such as West Kennet in Wiltshire and Maeshowe in Orkney, and often, as at Newgrange in Eire, the function of these structure is shown not to be for burials by the precise alignment of the passage to sunrise on a special day in the Celtic calendar. This astronomical function indicates that the barrows were in reality celestial observatories and that any burials, as in a modern cathedral, were by-products of the sanctity of the site, not the primary motives for construction. Like the later crypts of Christian churches, these passage structures were generally only semi-subterranean, below the artificial surface of the mound yet not fully below ground level. This may have had some ritual significance, and in the case of astronomical observatories was a functional necessity. About three furlongs from the south-eastern end of the Loch of Harray in Orkney stands the greatest of the Orkney

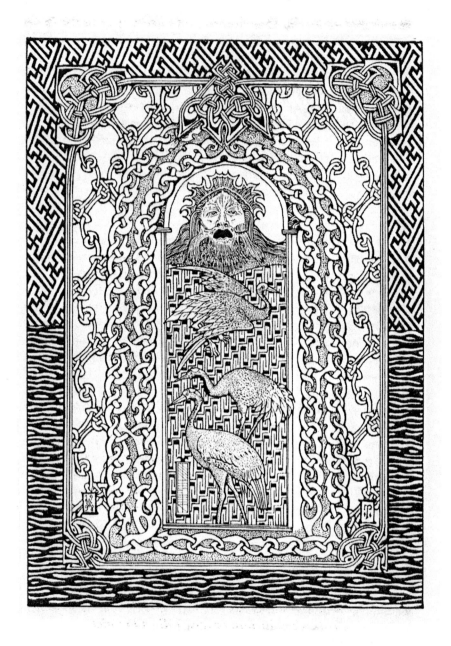

30

chambered mounds, Maeshowe. Outwardly, the howe is an earth mound about 115 feet in diameter and some 24 feet in height. Internally, the howe has several chambers at the end of an approach passage 54 feet in length. The main chamber is constructed of closely-fitted, levelled megalithic stones so well arranged that the jointing has been compared with that of the Great Pyramid at Giza. Above the main chamber, stones weighing three tons apiece are fitted together to make a corbelled vault, and connected to the chamber are three smaller subsidiary rooms.

The 54-foot passageway belies the claim that the howe was made solely as a tomb. It acts as a telescope-like sighting tunnel aligned upon a conspicuous standing stone 924 yards distant. This alignment is not chance, for it precisely defines a solsticial sunrise, astronomically linking the structure with the rotation of the heavens and the passage of the seasons. Another monolith to the west, called the Watchstone, marked equinoxes. Far from being sepulchral, the howe was an underground observatory used in an unimaginably distant period of history for the creation and monitoring of the calendar.

Such astronomical accuracy parallels the precision with which the stones were dressed. Archaeologists have determined that the chisels used to dress the stones were seven-sixteenths of an inch in width, which demonstrates two important facts about the ancient Orcadian workers: that their tools were standardized, and that the measures they used were related to the present Imperial System of measures still in use today in Britain and the United States.

---

3. Mider, Irish and Manx Lord of the Celtic Underworld, with his three guardian cranes. (Nigel Pennick

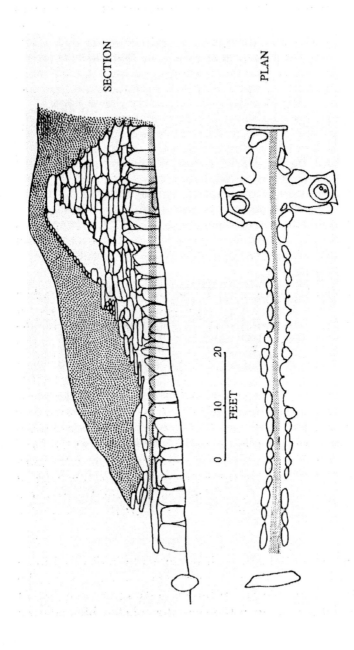

SECTION

PLAN

0   10   20
FEET

4. The 'passage-grave' at Newgrange, County Meath, Eire. Section and plan showing the solar orientation of the megalithic passage. (Nigel Pennick)

The orientation of subterranea upon important sunrises was also practised in ancient Egypt. The great temple at Abu Simbel, hewn in its entirety from the living rock, was made exactly according to the plan of the free-standing temples of Egypt, which were always oriented to important astronomical events. Inside the entrance are two subterranean courts supported by huge piers, and beyond are smaller chambers connected by galleries. At the far western end of the temple is the Holy of Holies with its images of the gods and King Rameses 11. This inner *sanctum* is penetrated by the rays of the sun on a special day in exactly the same manner as the passage grave at Newgrange in Eire.

A vivid description of this spectacular phenomenon has been left us by a correspondent to the *Pall Mall Gazette* of 20 April 1892:

The great temple is dedicated to Amen-Ra, the sun-god, and on two days a year the sun is said to rise at such a point that it sends a beam of light through both halls till it falls on the shrine itself in the very Holy of Holies. Mnay theories are based on the orientation of the temples, and Captain Johnston wished to find on which day in the spring of the year the phenomenon took place; so he took his instruments and we all went up to the temple before dawn. It was 26 February. The great hall, with its eight Osiride pillars, was wrapped in semi-darkness. Still darker were the inner hall and shrine.... a hard white light filled the sky. Clearer and whiter it grew, till, with a sudden joyous rush, the sun swung up over the low ridge of hill and in an instant .... one level shaft of light pierced the great hall and fell in living glory straight upon the shrine itself.

The incoming sunlight in such monuments is directed upon the sacred image at the precise moment of sunrise. At Abu Simbel it illuminated the tutelary deity of the temple. At Newgrange it shines upon the carved symbols which adorn a

stone at the far end of passage. Similar illuminations have
been observed recently in Arizona, and are well documented
from another religion which worshipped in hypogea -
Mithraism. In *Mithras- Geschichte eines Cultus*, M.J.
Vermaeseren says that Mithraic temples were frequently
oriented towards the east in such a way that the first rays of
the rising sun hit the representation of the bull-slaying god

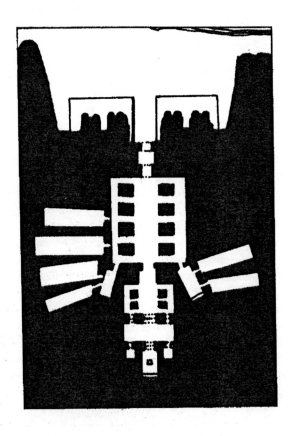

*5. Groundplan of the rock-cut temple of Abu Simbel, Egypt
(Nigel Pennick)*

through a window or other aperture in the vault. At Angera, the Mithraeum was a rock-cut hypogeum oriented so that the rising sun penetrated an aperture above the entrance to illuminate the main image. Where for technical reasons the whole hypogeum could not be oriented , the image was placed so that its illumination by the rising sun would still occur. The entrance to the rock sanctuary at Rozanec in the former Czechoslavakia was on the south side of a semi-circular

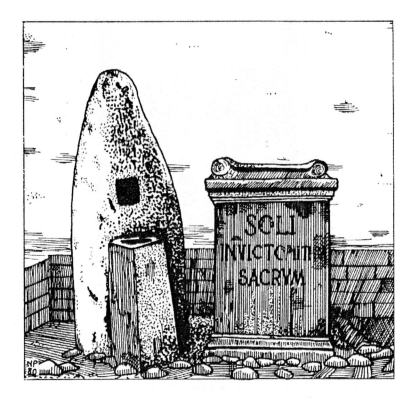

6. The Mithraeum at Spoleto, Italy, with triangular marble prism, standing stone and altar. (Nigel Pennick)

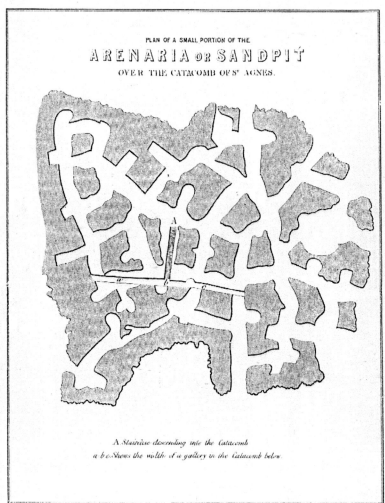

PLAN OF A SMALL PORTION OF THE

ARENARIA or SANDPIT

OVER THE CATACOMB OF S^T AGNES.

A Staircase descending into the Catacomb
a. b. c. Shews the width of a gallery in the Catacomb below.

London. Catholic Publishing & Bookselling Company Limited. T Booker, Manager. 35 New Bond S^t

36

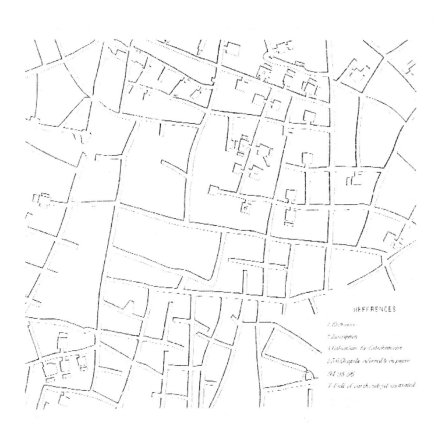

REFERENCES

7 & 8. The Catacombs at Rome, Italy. From J. Spencer Northcote's <u>The Roman Catacombs</u>, London, 1859. (Nideck)

37

chamber, but the image of Mithras was placed in the west so that it would face east.

In Mithrea, apertures were made in the roof at key points so that the sunlight could enter, and such 'light funnels' were made irrespective of the axial orientation of the shrine itself. In this respect they were a departure from the convential orientation of buildings where the whole axis of the structure is oriented towards some special sunrise, as, for example, in English medieval churches. Such an arrangement was more convenient for rock-cut shrines or crypt-like places, for natural apertures are more often than not oriented in some direction other than that required.

In addition to the image, other objects referred to as 'altars' were the focus of the sunlight from the light funnels. These 'altars' were in fact complex instruments of observation - gnomonic sun-makers. The Mithraeum at Spoleto in Italy contained a marble prism which had a hollow carved in its upper side. This was placed in front of a conical standing stone which had a square hole carved through it, and to the right of this megalith was an altar. If a gnomon were placed in the prism's hollow, a shadow was thrown into the square hole behind. Its function was probably timekeeping, for such a system of marking the passage of time by shadows is in use to this day at the Mosque at Isfahan in Iran where a gnomon indicates the time for prayers.

The Mithraic system of light funnels from the surface into underground places was adopted by the Christians who used identical systems in the Roman Catacombs. Of all ancient subterranea, these catacombs are perhaps the best known. 'The subterranean excavations in Rome,' wrote J. Spencer Northcote in *The Roman Catacombs* (1856), 'which are now known by the name of the Catacombs, may be briefly described as labyrinths of galleries hewn out of the living rock, crossing and recrossing one another in all directions, and here and there opening into small chambers of various shapes and sizes. They are rightly famed, not only on account of their association with early Christianity, but because of their antiquity and extent.

Some of the early Roman catacombs were re-used abandoned sand mines, but later they were excavated for the express purpose of burying departed Christian believers. Between the years 70 and 410 C.E. thousands of tunnels were built. Digging at first in secret, the *fossores* or diggers constructed a veritable subterraneaous city of the dead. As they expanded and filled with the remains of dead churchmen, so the new generation of Christians would enter the catacombs with the express intention of holding services at the tombs of these worthies. Various Pagan emperors issued edicts from time to time to prevent the adherents of this 'new superstition' from holding assemblies in, or even entering 'the places they call cemeteries'. On one occasion, when a band of Christians was seen entering the Catacombs to visit the graves of the martyrs Chrysanthus and Daria, the emperor ordered the entrance to be walled up with a mound of sand and stones, and the helpless worshippers were buried alive. This practice of clandestine worship in the Catacombs led the Pagan Romans to regard Christian devotees as aberrations - in the words of Minutius Felix, 'a skulking, darkness-loving race'.

The use of light funnels borrowed from the Mithraists helped a little to mitigate the darkness of the Catacombs. St Jerome, remembering his Sunday visits to the Catacombs as a boy, recounted that 'Here and there a little light, admitted from above, suffice to give a momentary relief from the horror of the darkness'. Prudentius, describing the Catacombs of St Hippolytus, wrote: 'As you advance further through the narrow and intricate passages, your progress is illuminated by an occasional ray finding its way through an aperture in the roof; so that, in spite of the absence of the sun, you enjoy its light far below the level of the ground. In such a place as this lies the body of St Hippolytus. ' Such apertures, arranged to illuminate the *archosolia* (burial niches) or the altars of underground chapels, are known as *luminaria*.

Rock-cut shrines like the Mithraea were not restricted to the Classical era or religions. Pagan medieval Europe also had its own traditions of sacred subterranea connected with celestial phenomena. In the vicinity of Detmold in Westphalia, the mystic heartland of Germany, stands a massive outcrop of rock known as the Externsteine. These three great rock pillars, which in mystical terms hold a similar position for Germans as Glastonbury does for the British, have been the focus of Germanic folk religion for millennia. Carved out of the summit of one of these rock pillars is a small chapel known as the *sacellum,* which has an altar and a curious circular window.

In 1823 the antiquary von Bennigsen studied this *sacellum*. He noticed that the circular window was oriented towards the position of the moon at its northern-most extreme, and, when viewed from the niche opposite, allowed the observer to see the point of summer solstice sunrise. This exciting discovery was virtually ignored until 1925 when the geomantic researcher Wilhelm Teudt visited the site. Between then and 1928, he took many observations and determined that the lunar orientation was marked by one of his *heilige linien* or holy lines - astronomical sighting lines which determined the siting of ancient shrines. This holy or ley line was connected with another which ran along the solar alignment and passed through a stone circle at Bad Meinberg to the north-east of the Externsteine.

Teudt believed that the *sacellum* pre-dated the Christian-ization of Saxony by Charlemagne in the year 772. His archaeological investigations showed that the *sacellum* had suffered deliberate damage at the hands of the Christians, who had levered away large rock slabs leaving two sides of the *sacellum* open to the air. One of these slabs, now lying at the bottom of the pile, weighed over fifty tons. After the year 1120, the monks of Paderborn finally converted the *sacellum* into a Christian chapel, but the altar was quite unsuitable for normal Christian observances. According to Teudt, this strange altar was designed expressly as a resting-place for a gnoman, and from this observation, he was led to search for further example. In his major work *Germanische Heiligtiimer (Ancient German Sanctuaries),* published in 1929, he wrote: 'A growing mistrust of the adequacy of previous research, and of the accuracy of its conclusions impelled me to make my own investigations ... The solar cult at the Externsteine was only a minor part of an astronomical cult which was centralized for the whole race, and which was based on extensive scientific

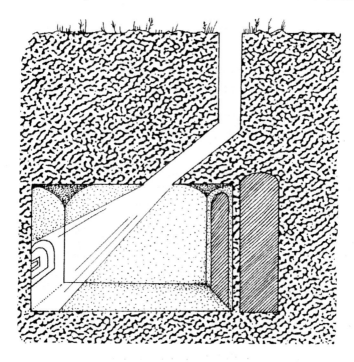

9. Chapel in the Roman Catacombs showing mode of operation of light funnel. (Nigel Pennick)

41

foundations.' His further studies led him to claim that a whole network of holy lines extended over Germany, a contention expanded upon by geomantic researchers such as Rohrig, Hopmann and Gerlach. Thus the rock-cut *sacellum* became the starting point of a whole school of geomantic research which flourished in Germany until the Second World War.

The majority of rock-cut shrines, chapels and monasteries have no such geomantic orientations, being cut into the most convenient rock faces. Some of the greatest sacred subterranea of antiquity fall into this category. In India, the most spectacular hypogea are the *chaityas* or underground temples. Vast spaces were excavated from the living rock in a style which reproduced in minute detail the wooden temples on the surface. Each and every architectural feature was carved directly from the rock, no building at all taking place. Some subterranea were of a vast size, those at Ellora alone extending to six miles of tunnel.

The earliest known rock-cut *chaitya* is in the Nigope Cave near Bihar, constructed in about 200 B.C.E. This *chaitya* is in the form of two halls, one rectangular in form 33 feet by 19 feet and the inner circular with a diameter of 19 feet. Later *chaityas* were of a more mature form, similar in plan to Christian basilicas. One near Poona has a forecourt, behind which is a space divided by columns into a nave and two aisles, terminating in a semicircular apse containing the shrine itself. This example penetrates the rock for a length of 126 feet.

The older *viharas,* or monasteries, were also rock-cut, and like their counterparts in Shropshire, Warwickshire and Yorkshire were divided into cells or chambers. Such *viharas* may have risen for several storeys into the rock, with interconnecting passages. The Kylas at Ellora is perhaps the finest, being richly carved in imitation of the finest Indian architecture of the period.

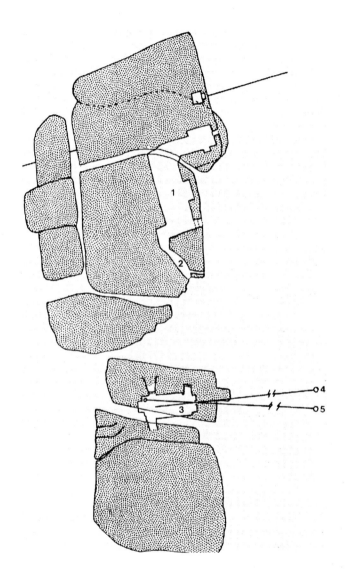

10. Plan of the Externsteine: 1. Central cave; 2. St Peter's Passage; 3. Sacellum; 4. Northernmost moonrise orientation; 5. Midsummer sunrise orientation. (Nigel Pennick)

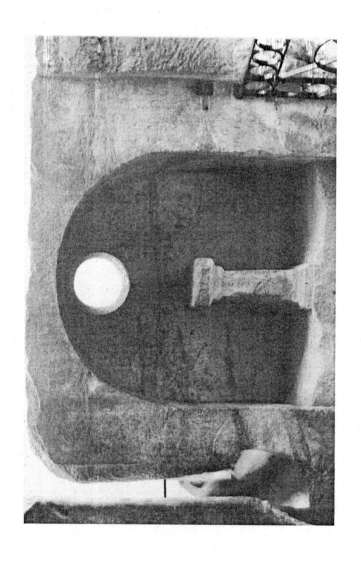

11. The Sacellum of the Externsteine, near Horn, Westphalia, Germany. (Nigel Pennick)

44

The remains of the rock-cut tombs and temples of the Nabataeans at Petra in Jordan are some of the most remarkable and beautiful subterranea in existence, outclassing even the Indian temples and monasteries. Complex and sophisticated Classical facades are hewn from the living rock and behind them extensive excavations penetrate the sandstone cliffs. Of many rock-cut monuments, the Khazneh Far'on- the so-called Treasury of the Pharoah - is the most impressive. Believed to be either the tomb of a Nabataean king, or alternatively a shrine of the Mother Goddess Allat, its Corinthian facade arises like a phantom palace amid the rough and unhewn cliff face.

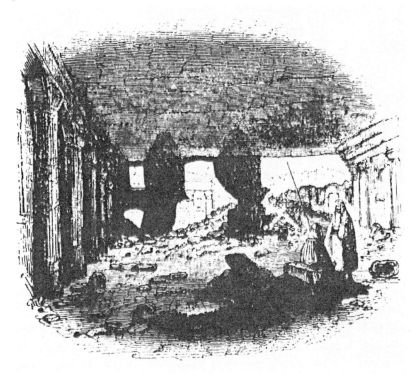

12. Interior of a rock-cut shrine at Petra (from Laborde's Sinai) (Nideck)

The deities of the Nabataeans, one of the three great pre-Islamic Arab civilizations, were closely allied with the Earth. The chief deities were Dushara and Allat. The former, a god, was symbolized by a block of stone or an obelisk, while the latter, a goddess, was associated with springs and water. Dushara was the tutelary god of the mountains into which Petra was hewn. His worship was intimately bound up with the solar cult of high places and standing stones, and in the third century rock-cut temple of Ed-Deir is a niche which contains a socket for the unhewn stone which symbolized Dushara. The worship of unhewn stones or obelisks in

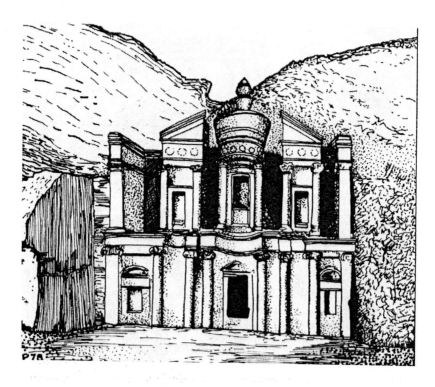

13. Ed-Deir, the rock-cut temple of Dushara at Petra, Jordan.
(Nigel Pennick)

hypogeal shrines has direct parallels in Mithraism and supposedly in the mysterious rites of the heretical Knights Templar.

When Christianity arrived at Petra, the zealots erased much of the ancient religion. At Petra, as in Greece, Rome and Egypt, the venerable temples were converted into churches. Near to the Ed- Deir shrine of Dushara are the remains of rock-cut Christian hermitages, and in the hypogeal temple itself a few small crosses carved inside tell their own tale of Christianization. The great era of magnificent rock-carving

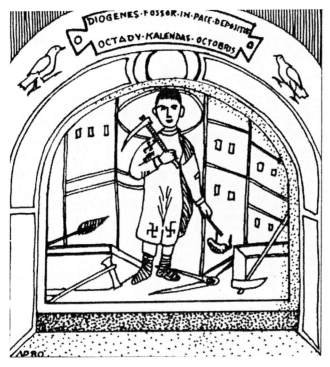

14. Early Christian miner of Roman times with lamp and pick. Swastikas on coat are magic sigils to protect the wearer from underground demons. From a painting in the Catacombs, Rome. (Nigel Pennick)

47

was now over. Small dwellings now called *Mughar el Nasara*, the dwellings of the Christians, were haphazardly carved into the cliffs in contrast to the canonical Classical art of the overthrown Pagans.

Complex underground shrines were made by Christians, however, but not at Petra. In former times it was the custom of the inhabitants of the Crimea to live underground for part of the year and the use of underground refuges in time of strife continued late. Before the Second World War, when the German occupation and Stalin's subsequent deportation of a large proportion of the populace disrupted the old pattern of life, the Crimea was famed for its flourishing rock-cut churches. Many of the shrines are unlike any other Christian buildings. They were not originally tombs, as is the case with Italian, Syrian and North Africa examples, neither were they monasteries like the Middle Eastern hermitages or the Indian *viharas*. One of the oldest was at Chekerman in the Crimea, 37 feet long by 21 feet wide, and but for the prominent cross which was obviously made as part of the original, its form could be mistaken for a Buddhist *vihara*. Beneath the fortress at Inkerman was a subterranean chapel similar to St Mary of the Rock in the Castle Rock at Nottingham in England, being a secure place for worship during times of siege. At Inkerman the chapel was connected with other subterranean rooms in precisely the same way as its Indian counterpart, indicating a monastic establishment. Close to Sevastopol was another underground church and monastery, and at Kieghart in Armenia is a similar hypogeum bearing the date 1288.

Underground places are natural repositories of chthonic powers, and as such many contain wells. Of course, many of these wells must have had purely practical uses, supplying subterranean monasteries and hermitages with essential water, but some certainly were ascribed healing or magical powers. A typical example is at Carreg Cennen, near Llandilo in mid-Wales where at the now-ruined castle, the legendary seat of Sir Urien, one of Arthur's knights, there is a subterranean well. Access is via a tunnel 150 feet in length, partly built and partly tunnelled through the rock. At the far end of the tunnel is a well which gives an unceasing flow of water, said to have curative properties. It was also an excellent insurance policy in time of siege.

Caves and Holy Wells

Subterranea can be places of human transformation. Those entering may emerge later as psychologically or spiritually changed people. Healing is dramatic a form of physical transformation, and local traditions tell how certain caves and tunnels possess healing powers. Water usually plays a key role in this, for many healing caves contain sources of water that function in the same way as curative holy wells. Caves created by dripping or flowing water often have pools of standing water inside them. Unusual shaped natural receptacles that catch and hold water dripping from above are often ascribed beneficial properties. A cave near Sanna at Ardmaurchan in the Scottish Highlands conains a water-filled rock basin whose contents are said to make people happy and strong.

Where they occur in a Christian context, it is likely that rock basins were used for baptism, another form of transformation. A cave near Campbeltown, reputed to have been the residence of St Kieran, contains a rock basin actually called St Kieran's Font. Its water is said to possess curative virtues. St Medan's Cave on the shore at Kirkmaiden near the tip of the Mull of Galloway in Scotland has an actual holy well inside it.

Rock basins are kept ever full by constant dripping from the cave's ceiling, and the uncanny clarity of sound that water makes when it drops into a subterranean rock basin seems to have the power to restore human abilities to make or receive sound. One such place is in another Scottish cave, the Dripping Cave at Craigiehowie, which is reputed to cure

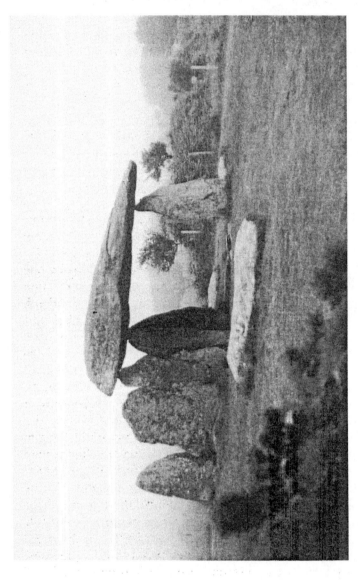

15. Pentre Ifan, near Nevern, Pembrokeshire, Wales. This megalithic structure, known as the "Womb of Cerridwen", said to be the last place where fairies were to between in Pembrokeshire, is reputed to be a gateway to the underworld. (Nigel Pennick)

deafness. The patient should lie on the cave floor and allow water from roof to drip into one ear, then the other.

Other subterraneous holy wells may have been the fore-runners of some major Christian cathedrals, for at Chartres, Glasgow, Nimes, Wells and Peterborough such wells were appropriated by the nascent church for its own use. Glastonbury Abbey's western crypt preserves such a well, to which access is gained from the crypt by a curious arrangement of staircases for entering and leaving pilgrims. It is not known whether this well was formerly sacred to the Old Religion, but it is believed to be fed by waters overflowing from the Chalice Well at the foot of Glastonbury Tor.

Although the Christian church appropriated the more important and obvious Pagan shrines, the country paganism of northern Europe literally went underground. In the Loire Valley of France, the old religion, proscribed in vain by the Church, was practised clandestinely in subterranea which were literally held to be the abodes of the spirits of the dead. Such rites may have existed in Britain, for it is recorded that the early Christian holy men of Scotland who frequented caves often had to exorcise their 'evil spirits'. In places where the power of the Church had increased, offerings for the dead were placed in pits rather than the actual subterranea. In other places, where the Church was less powerful or less observant, pits for offerings continued to be made inside the *souterrains*. In them are often found the remains of horses; their bones, skulls and even harnesses, as the horse was believed to be the transporter of the souls of the dead. Fragments of horse have been excavated from *souterrains* at Lumeau, Toury, Ruan and Selommes in Beauce north of Orléans. At Lumeau symbolic offerings were also found. These included eggs, stone balls, bone rings, whetstones, thimbles, fragments of pottery, blue stones and blue pieces of glass. All pottery in the pits had been broken as symbolic of death.

At the bottom of a funnelled-out pit at Toury, a complete horse skull was found placed on a flat stone and covered with a thick layer of broken pottery and miscellaneous animal bones. Horse bones and a skull were also found at Neuvy-en-Dunois at the junction of two galleries hewn in the rock. Here, ribs and vertebrae had been placed on a levelled bed of earth together with fragments of pottery which were dated to the fourteenth century. The whole deposit was covered with stones and surmounted by a horse's skull. In a *souterrain* at Ascheres-le-Marche, the complete skeleton of a horse was discovered, but interestingly, only three of its hooves were shod. This characteristic has been noted in many places in connection with the threefold lore of transition-points such as cross roads. From the threefold Roman god of the *trivium* to the English folk song *Widecombe Fair*, this 3 + 1 organization can be found. Its survival in Christian buildings like King's College Chapel in Cambridge demonstrates the pervasiveness of a little-studied numerological oddity.

The connection between subterranea and magic is long established; the abode of oracles and spirits, they were hence natural places of attraction to necromancers. Traces of medieval witchcraft have been found in many French *souterrains*. The jawbones of cats were discovered carefully arranged in a *souterrain* at Chameul's Farm at Chevilly, Loret, and at Châtres-sur-Cher, south of Blois, a strange *souterrain* of a sorcerer was excavated in the mid-1970s. Archaeologists found a very elaborate system of chambers, which in two places had been deliberately filled to prevent access to a western section which contained a Pagan *sacellum* and an even deeper cross-shaped gallery complete with altars. From this an even smaller creep gave access to yet another *sacellum* which contained a grave. At the entrance to the whole weird complex were various carvings including a detached head. Such heads were common cult objects in Celtic Pagan religion and have been found carved on geomantic rocks in Germany and in man-made subterranea in England,

Germany and the former Czechoslovakia. On the steps of the central altar of this secret *sacellum* were ten human images placed side by side with a nineteenth century oil lamp with its collar fractured. Most unusually, the souterrain at Châtres-sur-Cher is carved in clay, so it cannot be very ancient. This is forcibly confirmed by the date 1870 carved at the entrance of a side passage. During the last century the place was owned by a villager who had the reputation of being a 'cunning man',

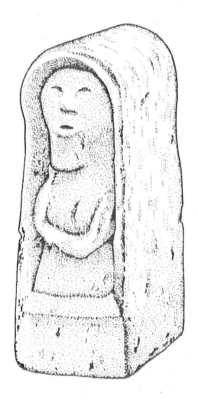

16. Votive figure from the souterrain at Châtres-sur-Cher, France. Height 2³/₄ inches. (Nigel Pennick, after Mauny)

so this *souterrain* is a remarkable survival of traditional underground Pagan religion into modern times.

That such secret rites should have survived past 1870 is even more amazing when we note that in 1226, following the inquiries of the Inquisition, the Council of Toulouse ordered that all *souterrains* in France suspected of being used by heretics were to be destroyed or filled in. 'Heresies' die hard, however, and during the sixteenth and seventeenth century a truly remarkable series of 'heretical' carvings was made in the *souterrain* at Deneze-sous-Doue, near Saumur. This cave, originally 52 feet in length, was partially destroyed by a roof fall during the eighteenth century and was not properly excavated until 1975 when a group of archaeologists under A. Heron found the extensive series of sculptures. Hundreds of carvings have now been brought to light. The Pagan nature of them is amply demonstrated by the human figures with animal heads which appear among naked men and women holding their genitals; processions; women breast feeding their babies; musicians with bagpipes and monsters or deformed people. A Pagan cult probably flourished here, as at Doute- la-Fontaine nearby, where Rabelais recorded 'devilries' or carnivals in which masked and costumed people took part. It appears that this *souterrain* was the hypogeum of the divinities in whose honour the 'devilries' were held.

Whilst French *souterrains* were the scene of clandestine Pagan rites, a more sinister use of underground spaces was used in nearby Germany for the suppression of such beliefs. The *Vehmgericht* or Secret Tribunal was a system of kangaroo courts whose purpose was the suppression of political and religious dissent. This peculiarly German institution was set up by Charlemagne after his conquest of Westphalia largely with the intention of suppressing paganism. The Vehmgericht, which met at ancient geomantic sites like mark-trees also practised their abhorrent judgements in subterranean vaults.

The offences with which the Vehmgericht was concerned were heresy, apostasy, sacrilege, witchcraft, rebellion, theft and robbery with Jews, adultery, rape and violence to women with child, and murder. The organization and rites of this tribunal were pseudo-Masonic. Eliphas Levi tells us in *The History of Magic* that 'The tribunal affected most fantastic forms of procedure: the guilty person, cited to appear at some disreputable crossroads, was taken to the assembly by a man dressed in black, who bandaged his eyes and led him forward in silence ... The criminal was carried into a vast underground vault, where he was interrogated by a single voice. The blindfold was removed, the vault was illuminated in all its depth and height, and the Free Judges sat masked and wearing black vestments.'

Such a vault exists beneath the Bergschloss, the upper castle of Baden. In 1824, James Skene wrote an account of these Vehmic subterranea, carefully arranged so that the maximum discomfort and terror could be experienced by the hapless prisoner before his judgement and inevitable execution. Of course, horrendous dungeons and torture-chambers existed and exist beneath virtually every major castle in Europe, for they were essential parts of the government of feudal society. The anti-heretical nature of the *Vehm*, like the inquisition, brings their subterranea within the realm of religious structures. However, the more agreeable view of sacred subterranea is that of quiet and holy places of contemplation, not the abject terror of the Secret Tribunal.

Breathing Caves

The European spiritual tradition sees caves as places of the breath of the Earth. According to human symbolism, caves represent the throat, and those where wind comes forth from the ground are seen as breathing-places of the Earth. There are a number of such places in the British Isles, all of which have been held in awe as sacred. Formerly, a cave called Breuant, 'The Windpipe' existed in Gwent, Wales. It was considered one of the Eight Wonders of Britain. Nennius describes it as "having wind blowing out of it constantly". Clement of Alexandria described the cave in his Stromata: "...in the island of Britain there is a cave situated under a mountain, and a chasm on its summit; and that, accordingly, when the wind falls into the cave and rushes into the bosom of the cleft, a sound is heard like cymbals clashing musically. And after, when the wind is in the woods, when the leaves are moved by a sudden gust of wind, a sound is emitted like the song of birds."

In Celtic spirituality, caves that make sounds like the singing of birds are said to be the dwelling-places of otherworldly birds. Irish and Manx traditions tell of the cranes of Mider that guard the entrance to the underworld. They tell passers-by to come no closer and to avoid being dragged in. Three monstrous demonic black bird called Cornu is said to inhabit St Patrick's Purgatory. The Goose is another Celtic cave-bird. Goose images in cave-art is known as far back as the Magdalenean era, and there are carvings of geese in Celtic caves, most notably in Fife, Scotland. Several British folk-tales about caves feature geese, who may be the sacred bird of Mother Earth. The goose appears as one of the archaic goddess-images of Old Europe, and in modern times as the doyenne of fairy-tales, Mother Goose.

Certain special caves are the source of mysterious noises; cracking and grinding, throbbing, booming and gurgling. Formerly, they were held in awe by locals and visitors alike. The twelfth-century writer Gerald of Wales tells of the wonderful noise he heard at a cave on Barry Island. He likened the rollling clash of the waves to otherworldly smiths labouring in the bowels of the earth. Bardic interpretations of cave sounds have likened them to the echoing notes of a bowed instrument, rumbling drums, droning bagpipes, howling dogs, wailing spirits and 'the good people's music'. In the Gaelic tongue, Fingal's Cave on the Island of Staffa is

56

called 'an Uaimh Binn', the Melodious Cave. Caves were chosen by sybils, bards and other spiritual people as places where they could listen to the natural breath of the Earth. Inside certain caves, sensitive people may sometimes hear intelligible voices. Certain caves are powerful places of oracular pronouncement, where the voice of the earth seems to speak to humans through the medium of inspired people. In the primal darkness of an oracular cave, the conscious mind is suppressed, and contact with elements of the unconscious can be achieved more readily than on the surface. The Cave of the Bard on the Orkney island of Bressay is such a place.

Underground places are very much places of breathing. In them, our own breath is at one with the chthonic breath. Human breath, called anadyl in Welsh Bardism, is seen as an aspect of this subtle cosmic breath that dwells within caves. Suffocation, losing the breath, is a fitting way to die in a cave, for underground structures can be lethal as well as inspiring. As in all things, the law of the unity of opposites is defined by a very fine line. When we enter a cave, we must breathe the breath of the earth, for good or ill. If this earth-breath is composed of noxious gases, then we will die.

Chapter Four

Hermitages And Crypts

Religious people following the contemplative life have often felt a need for solitude. The lives of hermits, anchorites and ascetics were often spent in isolation on remote islands, mountain-tops or in caverns underground. Natural caves were often chosen by the missionary ascetics of the early Church, especially in Scotland, where various caves still bear names which attest to their erstwhile use by religious men of antiquity. By Loch Kilkerran is St Kieran's Cave, at Wigtown, St Ninian's, and on Holy Island in the Clyde is the Cave of St Moloe, complete with runic inscriptions and incised crosses. St Adrian and his band of monks lived in a cave at Caplawchy in Fife, and the famous cave of St Rule at St Andrews was immortalized by Sir Walter Scott in *Marmion* (Canto I, 29), where he describes a 'palmer' or pilgrim who worshipped there:

> To fair St Andrews bound
> Within the Ocean cave to pray,
> Where good St Rule his holy lay
> From midnight to the dawn ofday
> Sung to the billows' sound.

On the foreshore a few miles from the monastery of Whithorn on the wild coast of Galloway, sixty miles west of Carlisle, is the cave of Physgyll. This is associated in the popular mind with St Ninian who used it as a retreat, described in an eighth-century poem from Whithorn as an *horrendum atreum,* an awesome cavern. Various Celtic crosses and grave-markers can still be seen. Whilst completely natural apart from a few inhumations and ritual niches, Physgyll is typical of the holy subterranea frequented by the ascetic British saints of the former Celtic Church. These caves, often haunted by malevolent spirits and ogres who were later personified in the cannibal Sawney Beane, often required thorough exorcism before their Christian occupants could take up residence.The cave of St Serf at Dysart required an especially thorough exorcism.

In an era of unbelief, natural caves made ideal refuges, but when the Church had been thoroughly established as an arm of the state, then public hermitages could be made without fear. Natural caves were still utilized, but hermits often felt it an act of piety to hew their own caverns into the living rock. Several ancient rock-cut hermitages still exist in Britain, some of them in a fine state of preservation. Most of the English rock-cut hermitages, having been made by the Saxons, are of the same type as those found in German-speaking Europe. At Bridgnorth, Staffordshire, the hermitage in the Rock of Atheardston has direct parallels elsewhere in Europe, having been made at a similar period, the tenth century.

Unlike churches, the chapels of rock-cut hermitages were not usually dedicated to specific saints. Where saints' names are connected with subterranea, the saint is often St Peter, 'The Rock'. The 'large cult-room' at the Externsteine has a connecting tunnel known as St Peter's Passage, and also in Germany near Goslar is the outcrop known as the Petersberg which contains a small rock-cut chapel. The connection with Peter comes not only from the utterance based on a pun on his name - the rock; the attribute of St Peter as holder of the keys of heaven and earth is appropriate for one connected with the underworld. The gatekeeper of the threshold of death is a Christianization of the many guardians of the entrance to the underworld.

One of the most important visions of St Peter was received in a rock-cut hermitage near Evesham in Worcestershire by the hermit Wulsi. During the reign of King Edward the Confessor he had a vision in which St Peter indicated the site for a most holy shrine near London: 'Fear not, brother: I am Peter, who keeps the keys of heaven. Tell Edward the king that his prayer is accomplished ... At London is the spot marked out,

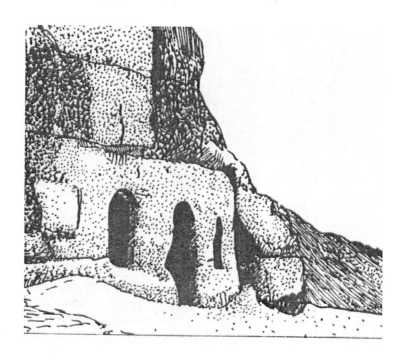

17. Rock-cut hermitage at Dale, Derbyshire. (Nigel Pennick)

60

two leagues from the city, at Thorney, where is a church, ancient and low ... towards the west on the Thames. I myself will consecrate the spot with my hands.' The visionary Wulsi wrote down the words of the apparition and had them taken

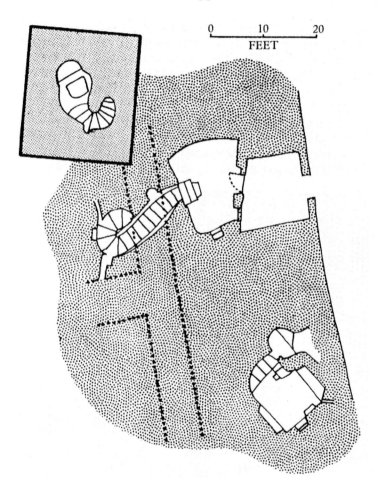

0   10   20
FEET

18. Underground hermitage at Pontefract, Yorkshire. Inset: lower level of stairs leading to water supply. (Nigel Pennick)

to the king, who duly founded the great Abbey of Westminster.

Rock-cut hermitages were often made in convenient crags near more ancient holy sites. The hermitage at Dale in Derbyshire, situated in a steep wooded hillside above the valley, guards the Hermit's Well, a sacred spring which never runs dry. Perhaps this was a Pagan holy well which was appropriated by the incoming Christian faith and needed a pious guardian to prevent the recurrence of Pagan worship there. Close to the church at Sneinton, now a suburb of Nottingham, was another hermitage cut in a low sandstone cliff. Near to this, and perhaps administered by the incumbent, were the holy well of St Anne and the unique turf maze which finally succumbed to the enclosure of common land at the end of the eighteenth century. Both of these sacred places were survivals of the old religion, as was a curious custom associated with two hermitages in Pontefract, Yorkshire. The hermit of the chamber hewn in the rock below Back Lane at Pontefract had to pay as his annual rental one white rose on midsummer's day, obviously a survival from pre- Christian days.

Even though the ancient rites of the Pagans slowly dwindled into folklore, the use of subterranea for healing and penance continued unabated, overseen by the watchful eyes of the local hermit, who was often in the pay of the local lord. According to the rules under which they placed themselves, only the barest necessities of life were allowed the hermit. Whilst the privations to which the hermit subjected himself were designed not to lead to physical collapse, the surroundings of the hermit were supposed to be as basic as possible as an aid to the contemplative life. The rock-cut hermitages fitted the bill perfectly. The only essential piece of furniture was held to be a crucifix upon which the attention and devotions of the anchorite could be focussed at all times. Such a crucifix, carved in the natural rock, exists in the anchorite cell carved at the foot of Cratcliffe Rocks near Stanton-in-Peak. The finest one known, it was adorned with budding foliage in its guise as the tree of life.

IRelanò

The most remarkable Celtic Christian sacred cave of them all is situated in Ireland on Station Island in Loch Derg. This otherworldly place was discovered in the twelfth century, when a knight named Owen spent a fortnight there in prayer and fasting. For the final night of his vigil, he discovered a cave, which he entered. During that terrible night, he underwent a spiritual transformation, in which he received visions of the afterlife. They were both heavenly and hellish. Returning to the world, Sir Owen related his experiences to Gilbert of Louth, a Cistercian monk from Lincolnshire in England. He spread the story among his religious order. The Cistercians identified Owen's visions with those of St Patrick. An episode in St Patrick's life tells how, on one occasion, he failed to convince his congregation of the existence of Heaven or Hell. So he prayed that God would show him a place where people could experience them directly. The Irish Apostle then discovered a cave in which people experienced visions.

The Cistercians believed that Sir Owen had rediscovered St Patrick's actual vision-cave, which was immediately re-named St Patrick's Purgatory. This Station Island cave rapidly became the object of Christian pilgrimage. The church put the Augustinian Order in charge of the cave, for it was considered too dangerous for people to enter it without supervision. Only those pilgrims who were deemed to be spiritually worthy, and who had paid the church for permission to enter, were allowed inside to experience the visions there, which seem no longer to have included the pleasures of Heaven, consisting only of demonic visions of the torments of Hell. Pilgrims were warned not to go to sleep, for, once one sleeps in the otherworld, one is lost to the world of the living. In the fifteenth century, people began to claim that the cave was losing its powers. So in 1497,

Rodrigo Borgia, Pope Alexander VI, declared the cave to be fraudulent and ordered its immediate closure. The guardians of the cave disobeyed the Pope, and in 1503, the Bishop of Armagh petitioned the next Pope, Pius III (Francesco Todeschini-Piccolomini) to grant indulgences for any who entered the cave. Pilgrims still visit the cave to-day, but unfortunately, it remains sealed.

A manuscript copy of *The Rule for Hermits,* dating from the fourteenth century and now in the possession of Cambridge University, says 'Let it suffice thee to have on thine altar an image of the Saviour hanging upon the Cross, which represents to thee His passion which thou shalt imitate, inviting thee with outspread arms to Himself.' Such rock-cut crucifixes also exist in the Royston Cave, at the Externsteine and in many Scottish subterranea.

Isolated outcrops of rock like the Externsteine, the Devil's Spittleful or Anchor Church at Repton were chosen as sites of especial importance. They were prominent landmarks, and as such were restored to by pilgrims, wayfarers, and those seeking penance for their sins. One such hermitage is at Guy's Cliffe near Warwick, a rugged precipice above the River Avon whose legendary occupier was Guy of Warwick. In the *Chronicle of Hyde Abbey* the tale of the semi-mythical vanquisher of the Dun Cow which laid waste Warwick is retold. Returning from a pilgrimage, the warrior arrived at Warwick, only to receive alms from his wife, who failed, to recognize him in his pilgrim's clothes. He then resolved to become a hermit and retire to a cave not far from his stronghold. Under the date 927, the story, recorded by the chronicler Gerard of Cornwall, reads 'He repaired to an heremite that resided amongst the shady woods hard by ... where he abode with that holy man till his death, and succeeded him in that cell.

The subterranean hermitage of Guy of Warwick is vesica-shaped about fourteen and a half feet long by five feet wide. An inscription, in a sort of runic script, generally believed to be fraudulent, was said to read 'Remove, O Christ, from thy servant this weight - Guthi.' Leland mentions the cave thus: 'Men shew a cave there in a rok hard on Avon ripe, where they say he used to slepe. Men also yet show fayr springs in a faire medow thereby, where they say that Erle Guido was wont to drinke.' The well, reached by a riverside path, has the never-failing flow typical of ancient sacred springs.

In the early thirteenth century, Brother Wiger, a canon of Oseney Abbey, went to live at the hermitage, having sworn a vow to live in solitude at the place called Gibbescliff. Another hermit, Gilbert of Warwick, described in an ordination list of 1283, probably lived there, but by the fifteenth century hermitages were on the decline. During the first year of the reign of Henry VI, Richard Beauchamp obtained leave to convert the hermitage into a perpetual chantry in which two priests would perform divine service for the souls of the founder and the king. The foundation was made as a votive offering to God to gain a male heir. Beauchamp had visited an anchoress (female hermit) at York, Dame Em Rawghtone, and received a prophetic utterance to the effect, carrying on the connections of prophecy and fertility.

In keeping with the increase in the wealth and complexity of the monasteries, by the late Middle Ages some hermitages became quite magnificent affairs. An example is the hermitage at Warkworth in the Avon Gorge, where the Chapel of the Holy Trinity, of three bays carved in the gothic manner, was constructed. This magnificent chapel was correctly oriented, with its altar at the eastern end. Such a chapel is reminiscent of the *sacellum* at the Externsteine, though it is illuminated from the west and south by elaborate decorated windows. In the recess to the south of the altar is a recumbent tomb effigy of an unknown female. In his *Survey of the Lands*

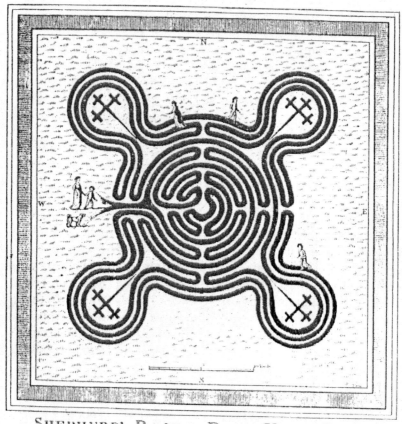

SHEPHERD's RACE or ROBIN HOOD's RACE,

A Maze or Labyrinth, its Site was on the Summit of a Hill near St. Anns Well,
about one Mile from Nottingham. It appear'd to have been cut out of the Turf
as a Place of exercise. Dr. Stukely supposd it of Roman Origin. Dr. Deering
imagind it more ancient than the Reformation, and made by some Priests
belonging to St. Anns Chapel, who being confind so as not to venture out
of Sight or Hearing, contrived this as a Place of Recreation. The Length of the
Path 535 Yards. On Inclosing the Lordship of Sneinton it was ploughed up
Feb. 27th 1797. — Published March the 27 1797, by J. Wigley Nottingham. —
Price Sixpence Plain. Eightpence Col----ed.

19. The maze formerly at the rock-cut hermitage and holy
well of Sneiton, Nottingham, England. Engraving by
J. Wigley, 1797. (Nideck)

of the Percies (1586), Stockdale writes: 'There hath been in the said parks one house hewen and wrought in a cragg or rock of stone, called the Harmitage, having in the same a hall, kytchen, chamber and chapell.' Here, life for the hermit must have been quite pleasant. He had a garden above the chapel, a byre in which to keep his cows, and was allowed pasturage for horses and cattle, receiving twenty marks a year and twenty loads of firewood. Once a week he was permitted to net salmon.

The relatively affluent life of the hermit contrasts strongly with the penitential and ascetic lives of the early hermits in their bare and cheerless caves. This contrast was all too apparent at the time of the Reformation, which dispossessed monasteries and hospitals, and suppressed hermitages. But although the hermits were driven out by the King's Commissioners, the hermitages were still desirable residences. Local people soon found them useful accommodation, and their new owners found them lucrative sources of income. A rental of 1591 records the fate of the Hermitage at Sneinton, Nottingham: 'The ermitage of Sneynton being a house cut out of rock and payeth yearly 2 shillings.' It is only within living memory that the last rock-cut houses, formerly the cells of anchorites, were vacated at Kinver Edge.

Women's Mysteries

Chthonic places have always been primarily associated with women's mysteries. Many ancient caves and tunnels have names that recall this tradition. In the Mendip Hills, near Leighton, Somerset, the White Woman's Hole recalls sybilline inhabitants. Sometimes, the female occupant was the horrid Morrigan, sometimes the Fairy Queen or the Queen of Elfland, and sometimes a human wise woman.. In traditional society, men resorted to such places to gain instruction. The Scotsman who learnt to play the bagpipes in a cave at Harlosh Point was taught by an otherworldly female. Just as

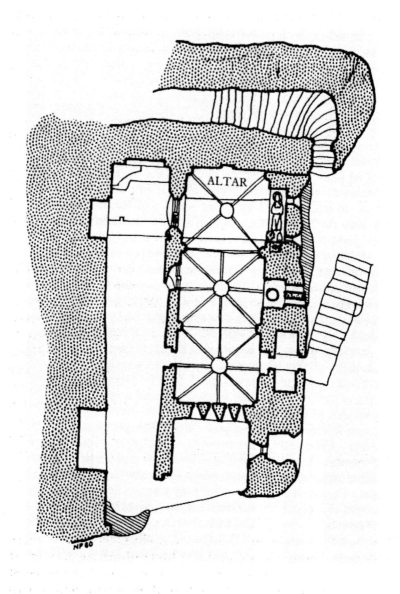

ALTAR

20. *Rock-cut hermitage, Warkworth, containing gothic chapel:*
plan. (Nigel Pennick)

Scottish highland bagpipers must use their breath to make music, so seeresses use their breath to pronounce oracles. The inspiration of musicianship as much as seership lies in the unconscious mind, which may be likened to the darkness within the Earth.

European sacred caves are places of mediumship. In England, the notable fifteenth-century soothsayer Mother Shipton lived in a cave at Knaresborough in Yorkshire, whilst in south Germany, in the side of the Teck, an ancient Celtic holy mountain, is the Sybillenloch. According to legend, this cavern was the seat of a benevolent woman who gave counsel to local people and made fields and flocks fertile by passing around them in her chariot pulled by cats.

A tale from the Dominican Order tells how a Roman Catholic spiritual practice originated in the feminine otherworld. According to the Breton Black Friar, Alain de la Roche, who flourished around 1470, the beads of the Rosary were received from the spirit-world in 1214 by the Inquisitor Dominico de Guzman. Having failed in his mission to convert the Cathars to Roman Catholicism, de Guzman went into retreat. In order to meditate, he entered a cave in a wood near Toulouse, an ancient Celtic holy place. After three days' penitential fasting, he experienced the apparition of the Madonna, three queens and fifty maidens. From them, he received the Rosary, which rapidly became an essential element of Catholic devotions, which it remains to-day.

Crypts

Many of the important places of early Christianity were subterranean. The legendary birthplace of Christ at Bethlehem was in a subterranean stable, and his place of sepulture was a rock-cut tomb in Jerusalem. These two places, with the addition of the Crypt of the Eleona at Jerusalem, the earliest sanctuary dedicated to the Ascension,

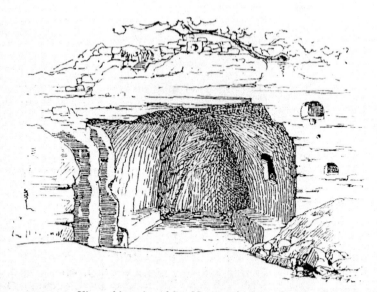

View of interior of St. Margaret's Cave, Dunfermline.

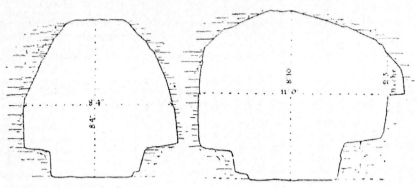

Sections of St. Margaret's Cave, Dunfermline.

21. St. Margaret's Cave, Dunfermline, Scotland. Drawing by F. R. Coles, 1897 (Nideck)

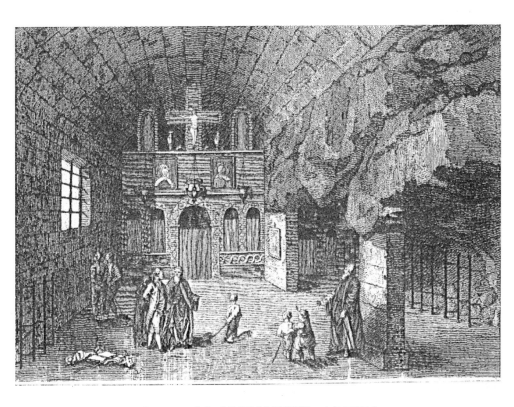

22. The Grotto of the Apocalypse on the Mediterranean island of Patmos, where St. John the Evangelist is supposed to have had his revelation. (Nideck)

71

were the three great 'holy grottoes' of the Holy Land. Above all three, elaborate and sumptuous churches were erected by the Byzantine emperors. The Church of the Nativity was built over the stable-cave; the circular Holy Sepulchre church, held to be the centre of the world, was erected above the tomb of Christ; and a massive shrine was constructed by St Helena over the grotto of the Eleona. In addition to these three, another important grotto in Jerusalem was held in reverence by Christians: the Chapel of the Invention of the Holy Cross. Here, according to tradition, the hiding place of the true cross of Christ was made known by divine revelation to St Helena. The cross, buried intact, was excavated from an underground structure which was thereby sanctified to become the fourth

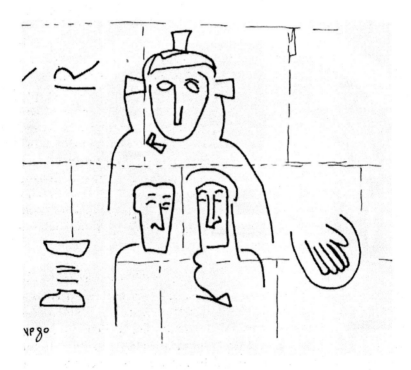

23, Graffito from the crypt of Rochester Cathedral, circa thriteenth century. (Nigel Pennick)

72

great grotto. The cross was later dismembered and parts of its spread all over the churches of Christendom.

With such a strong tradition of subterranean worship, reinforced by the extensive Roman Catacombs, it is not surprising that underground places of devotion have always played their part in Christian holy places. From the grotto of the Nativity to the Grotto at Lourdes, the faithful have descended into the earth to make their obeisances to the sacred personages of Christianity.

In many places it is certain that the crypts beneath present-day Christian shrines were originally of pre-Christian origin; several Mithraea in Rome were so adapted. In other places, the crypts were built as part of the original fabric; the Saxon crypts of England are examples of this. Five English cathedrals have easterly-situated crypts founded before the year 1085. They are all in old Roman towns: Gloucester, Canterbury, Winchester, Rochester and Worcester. The crypts are large in extent and underlie the most sacred parts of the cathedral fabric - the choir and (if present) the apse. Underlying the high altar they form, in effect, semi-subterranean churches set apart from the main body of the cathedral yet occupying the site of maximum telluric energy. As the positioning of sacred buildings was related to the energies circulating through the earth, the crypts, being half above and half below ground level, were areas of special closeness to these energies.

Like the crypt of Chartres Cathedral, which incorporated a pagan *sacellum* into its design, these early cathedral crypts were a reflection of the design of the churches above. The crypt at Gloucester Cathedral, for example, incorporates five apsidal side chapels below the original five ground-level apsidal chapels. Such reflected forms were a development of the earlier Anglo-Saxon crypts, which are perhaps the most intriguing pre-conquest structures remaining in England. At

Ripon, Hexham and Repton are three subterranean shrines, the first two of saints, and the latter of a king - Aethelbald of Mercia.

The crypts at Hexham and Ripon were arranged for the display and veneration of relics, being derived from the *confessio* of the early Roman basilicas, which was a chamber containing relics below the high altar, usually with an opening to the church. This aperture was generally in the direction of the congregation, supposedly for the beneficial rays emanating from the relics to bathe the worshippers in healing energies. In the crypts, access was by steps at each end for the progress of pilgrims past the displayed relics. The crypts at Hexham and Ripon were founded by St Wilfrid

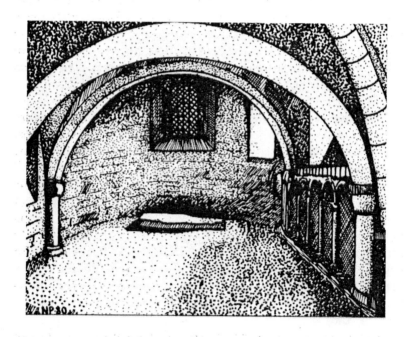

24. Side chapel in the crypt of Gloucester Cathedral. (Nigel Pennick)

before the year 678. Their orientation is the reverse of normal, which indicates a possible 'light funnel', but none has been observed. Bede recounts that Wilfrid was buried at Ripon 'south, next to the altar', which means in the crypt itself, so that shrine must have been for pilgrims visiting the sepulchre of the founder.

The crypt at Repton was a splendid mausoleum in which the body of King Aethelbald was laid to rest. As a representative of sacral kingship, a concept still very strong in Anglo-Saxon times, his remains were equally if not more powerful than those of the church's holy men. Befitting a royal mausoleum, the Repton crypt still retains its spiral columns. Columns of this form have always been reserved for places of exceptional sanctity. Triple spiral columns were used to support the roof of the shrine of the protomartyr of Britain, St Alban, at the city which bears his name. The *baldaccino* of St Peter's in Rome is likewise held up on pillars which, in tradition, originated in Solomon's Temple at Jerusalem, and indeed it is the famous temple which was the masonic prototype for spiral pillars.

Just as the most sacred Christian shrines of Palestine were subterranean, so with the holiest places of other countries. The most sacred Christian shrine in England is at Glastonbury and this, too, has both a system of tunnels and also a crypt. Like many things in Glastonbury, this crypt is out of the ordinary, for both its situation and its late date of construction render it unique. At present, much of the crypt is actually open to the exterior, yet originally it was totally subterranean in character. Unlike the common Norman crypts which are only half, or at most, two-thirds, below ground level, that at Glastonbury was dug to a great depth so that the crown of the vault is level with the ground.

The situation of the crypt, too, is like no other, being excavated beneath the Galilee porch and St Mary's Chapel at the west end of the Abbey buildings, and communicates with

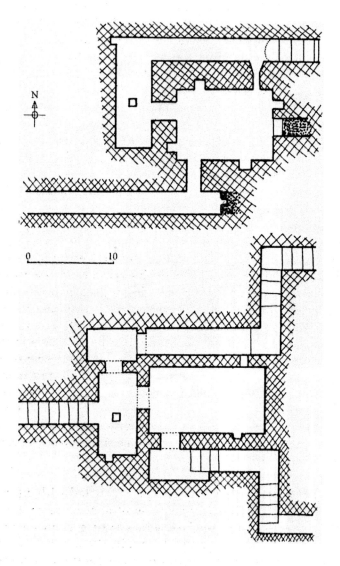

*25. The Anglo-Saxon crypts at Ripon and Hexham: plan.
(Nigel Pennick)*

a well reputed to be filled from the Chalice Well further east. This Galilee crypt was first excavated as late as the year 1500, and was built in two stages: firstly, beneath the Galilee, then later extended below St Mary's Chapel itself. The architecture of the crypt is odd, the masons having simply re-used some old Norman vaulting ribs and constructed new vaults from ancient materials, perhaps with the intention of lining a most sacred site with material already hallowed with centuries of use. When this was complete, the excavation westward was made and the vaulting completed in the most modern style - perpendicular.

At some time after the Dissolution, the crypt was filled in with earth. For centuries it lay forgotten, but in 1825 a Mr Reeves noticed some steps. Curious, he began to dig, and his diggings took him fifteen yards north, below the present footpath, at which point he discovered eighteen wooden coffins. In 1826 Reeves cleared the crypt of its earth filling and in so doing also rediscovered the well. It is approached by a passage fifty feet long of which only the entrance was known before Reeve's excavation. It was made at the same time as the crypt, and, like the main body of the crypt, is vaulted in perpendicular style. The well itself seems much older, perhaps pre Christian and the original cult-object at Glastonbury in association with the mysterious egg-stone which now leans against the Abbot's Kitchen. The actual function of the western crypt is yet to be determined. Like many of the mysteries of Glastonbury Abbey its abnormality indicates some use peculiar to the site.

Most modern churches have been constructed without regard to the ancient canonical practices of sacred geometry, and their sites chosen by cost exercises rather than geomancy. Guildford Cathedral, however, begun in 1936, was constructed according to the correct canonical principles. Its siting, orientation and sacred geometry are determined according to the age-old geomantic principles. Below the majestic cathedral, which stands atop Stag Hill above the town, there is a series of tunnels and a crypt in addition to the more prosaic oil-fuel tank house, heating chamber, lavatories, chair store, organ-blower and cleaners' rooms. A cross tunnel connects the heating chamber on the north side with the organ blower on the south, and a longitudinal tunnel runs from the east end to the crossing beneath the tower where

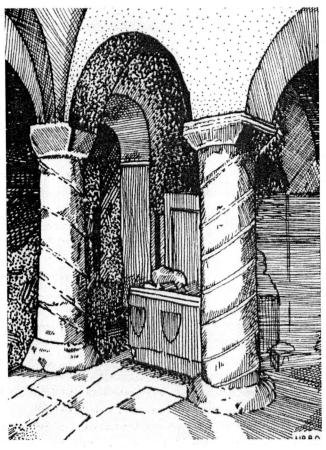

26. The crypt at Repton, originally the mausoleum of the Saxon King Aethelbald of Mercia. The spiral 'Solomonic' pillars show the sanctity of the shrine. (Nigel Pennick)

another transverse tunnel crosses it on the centre-line of the tower. This central tunnel has three branches with creeps running to important points of the building's substructure. Whilst the tunnels may be only for inspection, their positioning is exactly in the positions where a dowser would find patterns beneath a medieval cathedral, so they may serve some more esoteric function as well.

Although many royal personages and even whole dynasties are interred in cathedrals and mausolea all over the world, one of the most remarkable burial crypts is without doubt the Pantheon of the Kings at the monastery of El Escorial in Spain. Built directly beneath the high altar of the basilica, the Pantheon of the Kings is an octagonal crypt thirty-four feet in diameter lavishly decorated with fine marble and jasper from Tortosa and Toledo. Constructed to contain the bodies of the Spanish kings, the last burial was as recent as 1980 when the previous king was brought back to be re-buried among his ancestors.

The founder of El Escorial, Philip II, wished to build a Pantheon beneath the high altar, but he died before it could be started. His son, Philip III, wishing to fulfil his father's vow, commenced work in 1617 under the direction of the master architect Juan Gomez de Mora. The work began with Pedro de Lizargarate as contractor, and after only two years the work was complete. But by 1621 the king was dying and a massive spring arose in the crypt directly beneath the high altar. This flooded the crypt completely, and the Pantheon was not drained until 1645 when Fr Nicolas de Madrid remedied the problem. It was finally consecrated in 1654 by Philip IV. The welling-up of a spring beneath the high altar demonstrates its geomantic siting, as many important points in cathedrals and monasteries have been shown by dowsers to be positioned over powerful blind springs, and at El Escorial this was verified the hard way.

Perhaps the most sinister crypt of modern times was that built on the express orders of Reichführer-SS Heinrich Himmler, the most feared man in Nazi Germany. Himmler's obsession with the occult is well known, but less well documented is his interest in geomancy and sacred geometry. Through the *Ahnenerbe*, a research organization set up to investigate all aspects of ancient German history and lore, Himmler accumulated a corpus of material on the *heilige linien* (ley lines) of Germany and the eastern 'empire'. Expeditions were dispatched to remote Tibet to establish the whereabouts of the mythical subterranean kingdom of Agharthi whilst others pored over the geometry of medieval Jewish cemeteries in the heartland of Germany. Himmler directed this research from a medieval castle rebuilt at enormous cost into a shrine to Naziism. Like other geomantic seats of political and spiritual power, Schloss Wewelsburg in Westphalia was triangular in form (the Kremlin and Westminster complexes are also triangular). It contained a vast hall in the middle of which stood a round table with thirteen chairs. In Arthurian manner, Himmler and his twelve *Obergruppenführer* Knights of the Black Order of the SS occupied these chairs. There, they would meditate in attempts to psychically influence Germany.

Beneath this reproduction Arthuriana was Himmler's mysterious crypt. Known as the Realm of the Dead, it was walled with stone five feet thick. The Holy of Holies of the Black Order, it contained a well-like cavity reached by a flight of steps. In the centre of this depression stood a stone stoup. In the event of an *Obergruppenfuhrer's* death, his coat of arms was to be burnt in the stoup and its ashes placed upon a pedestal in a niche specially provided for that purpose. Typically, four vents in the ceiling of the crypt were scientifically arranged so that the smoke would rise to the ceiling in a single column.

The Realm of the Dead was reputed to be the future mausoleum of Adolf Hitler himself, but events proved otherwise. Like the initiatory hypogea of antiquity, this mystic crypt was reserved for a chosen elite. It is fitting that the hyper-elitist Nazis should have as their central shrine such a traditional symbol of mystic initiation.

One might imagine that the Nazis were the last people to produce mystic subterranea, but that is not the case. Of all the rock-cut churches and mausolea in the world, the largest and most grandiose is that built in Spain on the orders of the Falangist dictator Generalissimo Franco. The Valle de los Caidos (Valley of the Fallen) in the Guadarrama Mountains north of Madrid is one of the few grandiose schemes of modern times to come to fruition. Hitler's great domed hall in Berlin and Peron's pyramid mausoleum of Eva were never built, but *El Caudillo's* huge subterranean basilica exists today. Hacked from solid granite by republican, communist and anarchist prisoners who had fought on the losing side in the Spanish Civil War, a vast underground cathedral was fashioned. Consisting of a vast domed area, only slightly smaller than the largest in Christendom, St Peter's in Rome, the subterranean cathedral contains a crypt and four *ossoria* or charnel-houses containing the bones of thousands of war dead.

Franco himself approved the ground-plan and siting of this unique house of the Falangist dead of the Civil War, and in 1959, the remains of one of the founders of Fascism, José Antonio Primo de Rivera was reburied with great pomp and ceremony in the mausoleum. Franco himself was buried here by a golden altar in 1975, flanked by the legions of the dead. Above his shrine a vast stone cross over 500 feet high was erected, illuminated at night to be visible from five Spanish provinces.

The siting of Franco's mausoleum is perhaps the last act of state geomancy carried out in Europe, for the vast underground basilica is sited at the centre of a cross formed by the lines between the cathedral at Avila and the Pantheon Condesa de la vega del Pozo; and Segovia Cathedral to El Escorial. The burial of the founder of a 'new order' at his country's *omphalos* or geomantic centre is an age- old concept, but seemingly out of step with the modern materialist age.

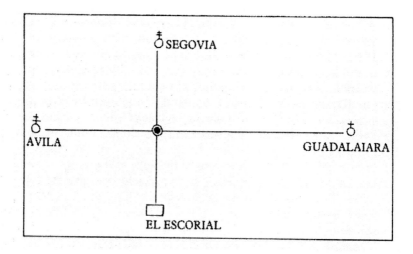

27. *The geomantic positioning of the Basilica of the Valle de los Caidos, tomb of Generalissimo Franco at the centre of a westward-facing Christian-type cross defined by the shrines at El Escorial and Guadalajara and the cathedrals of Segovia and Avila.*

Chapter Five

Unusual Uses of Subterranea

Many ingenious uses have been found for subterranea beyond the more obvious uses for transport, burial and religion. The enclosed nature of subterranean structures makes them ideal secure places for storage, refuges, prisons, factories and even dwelling-places. The ingenuity of people in modifying their environment to their advantage is amply demonstrated in the subterranean kingdom.

Underground Living Quarters

Although the slave miners of ancient Egypt and Rome were forced to live permanently below ground, many people have through preference chosen to become troglodytes. The Cimmerians, priests attending the subterranean oracles of the Classical world, made their habitation deep in the tunnels, as recorded by Ephorus (*circa* 500 B.C.E.): 'They live in underground dwellings which they call argillae, and it is through tunnels that they visit each other, back and forth.' The Cimmerians, like many monastic orders before and since, lived in rock-cut cells from which they emerged only to minister to the pilgrims visiting their shrine. At Baiae, the *argillae* of the Cimmerians surround the caverns of the Oracle of the Dead. The Cimmerians had a rule that they should never see daylight, so they never went outside the tunnels except at night, returning before dawn. Such a way of life is now traditionally ascribed to ogres and vampires.

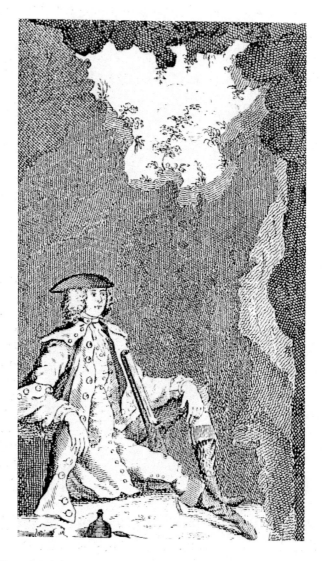

28. Certain subterranea are associated with outlaws. They include the notorious highwayman, Dick Turpin, shown here in his cave. (Nideck)

Pits with vertical entrances were once a popular form of dwelling. The Satarchae, the indiginous inhabitants of the Crimea, lived in them, and Xenophon noted that the Armenians also lived in well-like homes. Similar places existed in Britain, for during the last century a Mr Adlam discovered a series of pits near Highfield, a mile south of Salisbury, where, on a high chalk ridge between the Nadder and Avon valleys, prehistoric people had made their homes. The archaeologist E. T. Stevens examined over a hundred of these pits, which varied in depth from seven to fifteen feet, their internal widths ranging from six to twelve feet. The entrance was by a vertical circular shaft and the interiors were likewise circular. Stevens and Professor Boyd Dawkins in the book *Early Man* considered these of a neolithic date, though other researchers have thought them Bronze Age.

The Highfield subterranea were peculiar in that they had covers made from clay based on a framework of wattles which rested on ledges about a foot from the top of the shaft. Underground, the chambers were connected to one another by small apertures large enough for a person to creep through. People in remote parts of the Himalayas still retreat into similar structures for the duration of the winter, so it is likely that the Highfield subterranea also served that function. In the pits, the remains of food debris, especially split bones, indicates habitation. Among these split bones were human skeletal remains, marked in exactly the same way as those of oxen, horse etc., showing that these prehistoric troglodytes were cannibals. Perhaps such pit-dwelling cannibals are the origin of the ogre legends of ancient times and the prototype for H. G. Wells's morlocks of the *Time Machine*.

The earth houses of Scotland and Ireland, the *souterrains* of France and the Erdstalle of Germany were another type of subterraneous dwelling, used in some places as late as the nineteenth century. The Scottish earth houses are dealt with below. Rock-cut dwellings afforded greater comfort than pit-dwellings and survived into modern times. In an article titled 'Modern Troglodytes' published in *The Reliquary* in 1865, Robert Garner wrote: 'In this article we would especially bring before the reader instances where whole communities live in subterranean villages, and in our own times, and in Mid-England. The New Red Sandstone is particularly tempting for the formation of such dwellings, and was thereto excavated very largely in former times, for instance at Sneinton, and on the Lene in Notts. Also the lime debris near Burton, has been burrowed for the same object.'

In 1865 whole 'troglodyte villages' still existed in south-west Staffordshire and adjacent Worcestershire. The largest remaining village still inhabited in Garner's time was at Dunsley Rock, known locally by the nickname Gibraltar, where seventeen separate dwellings housed forty-two people. Several other rock-cut 'tenements' nearby were used as byres or styes. On enquiring of one troglodyte woman how many lived in her cave, she answered 'Nine of we', and told Garner that the rent for such a rock-cut dwelling was three shillings a week. Finally, 'We were satisfied with what we had seen of the troglodytes, without feeling any strong desire to become a member of any class of them ourselves.'

One of the last troglodyte villages in England was at Burton in Derbyshire, where the famous 'lime houses' existed. Here, in the spoil heaps from the lime-burning industry, the local lime workers burrowed mean dwellings. These impressed a French geologist, Faugas de Saint-Fond, who visited Buxton in 1784 and left the following account 'I looked in vain for the habitations of so many labourers and their numerous families without being able to see so much as one cottage when at length I discerned that the whole tribe, like so many moles, had formed their residences underground. This comparison is strictly just: not one of them lived in a house.' The lime houses were not pleasant places to live. 'Wretched and disgusting are these caves in the extreme', wrote one correspondent in 1813, 'and but for having their entrances closed by a door might be more easily taken for the dens of wolves or bears than the abodes of humanized beings.'

These vile hovels still existed as late as 1928. J. A. Goodacre, writing in *Buxton Old and New* published in that year stated that a fair specimen of those tenements still existed at the top of Duke Street, Burbage. Nellie Kirkham, a recorder of local lore wrote in 1947 that a man then aged seventy had been brought up in one of the lime houses. Fortunately they have now been relegated to the annals of the industrial revolution.

Prisons

Such appalling dwellings were used out of necessity for the lime workers were low paid and scarcely better than slaves. Similar underground places have been used more generally for punishment, and subterranean lock-ups were formerly quite common. Either purpose-built or converted from other disused structures, these lock-ups went under the curious name of *matamores* or *mortimores,* a word derived from the Arabic *matmuret,* a subterranean granary or crypt, cognate with the Arabic *muzmer,* a hiding place. In *Marmion,* Sir Walter Scott alludes to the *mazmorra* or prison beneath Crichton Castle. He claimed that the word *mazmorra* was brought back to Scotland by crusaders or merchants from the Near East. Such subterraneous prisons existed there, for it is recorded in the Biblical *Book of Jeremiah* that the unpopular prophet was cast into such a prison from which he had to be rescued, 'So they drew up Jeremiah with cords, and took him out of the dungeon.' This indicates that matamores used in Palestine were deep pits into which there was no access except by rope or ladder, perhaps being the remnants of ritual sacrificial shafts. In an era when human sacrifice had been discontinued, the capital punishment of prisoners had not been abandoned, and such matamores were just one slow and cruel method of execution.

Refuges and Shelters

Underground structures have always made useful refuges in time of war. Throughout history people have descended into the subterranean kingdom to escape from their enemies. During the Tartar invasions of the Crimea, the people retreated into their subterranea and remained safe from their depredations; the Anglo-Saxons are reputed to have fled underground to avoid the Danes; the earth houses of Scotland and Ulster show signs of having been refuges, whilst shelters have become a major feature of modern warfare. During the 1793 Royalist uprising against the Republicans in France there was extensive use of subterranea. 'In the eighteenth century wars of La Vendee', writes Ann Pennick in *Deneholes and Subterranea* '... in the forest of Meulac in Morbihan, 8000 men hid in an underground labyrinth. There was also a similar labyrinth in the Wood of Misdon, also in Brittany, where a secret society called *The Great City* hid from the French army.'

Such places are fine when undetected. Once discovered by the enemy, they become death-traps. In modern warfare, underground bunkers have often become tombs when poison gas or blazing petroleum from flame throwers has been pumped in through a discovered entrance.

Any underground structure, whether purpose-built or not, can be pressed into use in wartime. The Polish film *Kanal* retells the story of the heroic resistance against the Nazis in 1944 when urban guerrillas in Warsaw made extensive use of the sewer system. Sewers, cellars, natural caves and underground railways have all served in modern times as shelters from aerial bombardment, but during World War II special deep shelters were built in several British cities to augment the shallow shelters and re-used subterranea. The most notable of these are the New Tube Shelters.

In the journal *The Engineer* for the year 1942 is an account of these intriguing New Tube Shelters. On 3 November 1940 the Home Secretary had broadcast on BBC radio explaining that 'a new system of tunnels linked to the London tubes should be bored and tunnelling authorized in the provinces, where, with the aid of natural features, this could be done economically.' In response to this, London Transport was given finance to build deep shelters at ten sites. Two were found to be inconvenient for technical reasons, and shelters were finally constructed at Clapham South, Clapham Common, Clapham North, Stockwell, Goodge Street, Camden Town and Belsize Park on the Northern Line of the tube system and at Chancery Lane on the Central Line. Between 1200 and 1400 feet in length, the shelters were twin tubes sixteen and a half feet in diameter driven beneath the platforms of existing underground stations. Lying between 75 and 130 feet beneath the city streets, access was gained to the shelters by shafts which contained spiral staircases. The places chosen were arranged so that the shelters could be connected after the war to form new express underground railways for main-line trains, and plans were published in 1946 and 1949 incorporating the New Tube Shelters for this purpose.

Each shelter was divided into two levels and provided with bunks for sleeping, 800 per shelter. An ingenious double spiral staircase gave access near each end of the shelter, one turn for the top, the other for the lower level. Designed to accommodate 2000 people, each shelter contained eight lavatory tunnels, canteens, medical facilities, fail-safe power supply and no fewer than three alternative telephone systems for officials.

The shelters were complete by 1942, but were not open to the public until 1944 when the V-bomb attacks on London commenced. Three of the shelters were never open to the public, remaining in government hands for essential civil servants. At Goodge Street, the shelter was reserved for

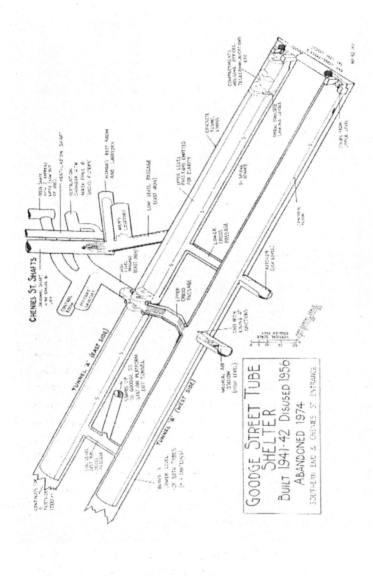

CHENES ST. SHAFTS

TUNNEL A (EAST SIDE)

TUNNEL B (WEST SIDE)

GOODGE STREET TUBE
SHELTER
BUILT 1941-42 DISUSED 1956
ABANDONED 1974
SOUTHERN END & CHENIES ST ENTRANCE

29. Diagram of part of the World War II underground bunker beneath Goodge Street tube station, central London. It is now used for the storage of security archives. (Nigel Penick)

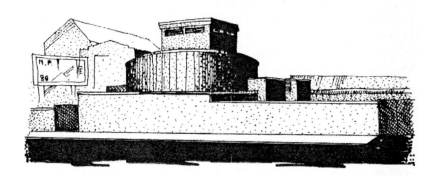

30. One of the entrances to the New Tube Shelter at Clapham South, London. The cubic compartment on top housed filters for poison gas, whilst the circular superstructure was the entrance to the spiral staircase. (Electric Traction Publications)

General Eisenhower and his staff. After the war, the New Tube Shelters were used for various purposes, but the new tube railways did not materialize. By 1951, the shelter under Chancery Lane station, originally intended as part of a tube from Camberwell to Euston, had been converted into a underground telephone exchange called Kingsway, which remained secret until 1972, when, to everybody's amazement, details were published in *The Post Office Courier*. Most of the New Tube Shelters are now abandoned, though security archives are stored in that at Belsize Park and the Camden Town shelter is used regularly by the BBC for 'futuristic' sets in television science-fiction series.

Military refuges in time of war are major engineering works in their own right. The vast bunker systems of the Maginot and Siegfried Lines and the later works of the German *Organization Todt* still exist in fragments large enough to show the special character of the new subterranea. As fire-power increased, so did the size and depth of bunkers, culminating in those fit to withstand nuclear attack. Perhaps the most extensive of these is the vast complex beneath Cheyenne Mountain in Colorado, where the computers and control centre for the United States in World War III are situated one third of a mile deep. The personnel accommodation at this and other US bunkers is a subterranean multistorey concrete building supported on vast springs to enable it to take the impact of a direct hit with a nuclear weapon. It is a frightening thought that the only survivors of the next war might be these present-day troglodytes.

Manufacture

The use of subterraneous factories is quite ancient. Apart from flintknapping *in situ* in the ancient neolithic flint-mines, the medieval use of subterranea for the malting and tanning industries is well- documented, especially in Nottingham. That city was renowned throughout England for the fineness of its beer because the many underground maltings in that town ensured a regular supply regardless of the season. Unlike surface maltings, those beneath ground level were kept naturally at a constant temperature, just right for the production of malt. The deep rock-cut cellars which still exist beneath the Salutation Inn and other old public houses in the city provided optimal conditions for the storage of beer.

At Edge Hill on the Liverpool and Manchester Railway, opened in 1830, the navvies dug underground locomotive sheds and maintenance facilities into the rock whose famous cutting provided a dramatic image for many an engraver. Dingy and sulphurous, these underground works are the ultimate in the 'dark satanic mills' image of the industrial revolution. They presage the 'sulphurous caverns' of the smoke-filled Metropolitan Railway of London 33 years later.

Underground factories in the modern sense came into being in Britain in the 1940s as a means of avoiding aerial bombardment. The new underground railway beneath Wanstead and Redbridge in east London was complete but without tracks when war broke out in 1939, so it was modified as an underground factory making vital aircraft components. Several similar factories were built elsewhere in Britain. One article in *The Engineer* for 1942 describes such an underground factory 'somewhere in England'. Begun in 1941 to house an aircraft components factory, the cavern system was cut through the rock leaving pillars to support the ceiling. Galleries over 1000 feet in length were shown, containing a two-storey underground administration office and concrete facings. As it is unlikely that new excavations were made, from the appearance of the tunnels this was probably in the abandoned workings of the Bath Stone Mines at or near Corsham in Wiltshire. Its exact location can only be guessed, as obviously it was not given for security reasons.

Storage

Almost every town in any country will have buildings with cellars, for underground storage is cheap and secure. Excavation of cellars is often simpler than surface building, and in places where the underlying geology is favourable, shopkeepers have dug extensive cellars into the bedrock. Cellars may be considered mere extensions of buildings, but underground storage away from buildings is of a completely different character. The use of underground pits with vertical entrances for the storage of grain is a specialized example of subterranea constructed away from buildings. Grain-pits of this type were once very widespread in Europe, North Africa and India. Until the last century, grain was stored in pits in the Touraine and Louret districts of France and in Spain their use dates back to antiquity. Varro and Pliny both mention the Spanish grain-pits, which were in ancient times either scattered or in small groups and in modern times dug beneath the streets of towns. In Barcelona there were fifty-nine pits surrounded by a wall at one location, and groupings of that many were not uncommon.

The typical grain-pit was a shaft thirty or more feet deep with a chamber at the bottom, similar in form to the deneholes of Essex and Kent, though it is hotly disputed whether these English examples were chalk-pits, refuges or granaries. However, at least one instance of a vertical-shafted grain store has been found in England, during the last century in a field called Wellhill at Peckham, then in Surrey, where there 'were the evident remains of three large wells, thirty- five feet in circumference. They had become choked up, but the occupier of the field had the rubbish cleared out of one, when he found the sides very nicely covered with smooth cement, and at the depth of about forty feet he came to a floor of lattice-work, resting on large upright timbers, and on the floor some straw.

'This floor completely filled the well, so that it is evident that it was not sunk for water; it seems to have been designed as a granary.' (*The History of Surrey,* Manning and Bray.)

Subterranean storage is ideal for valuables, and the vaults of banks are perfect examples of this type of structure. They are believed to have originated during the English Civil War when an enterprising shopkeeper in Nottingham used a rock-cut cellar beneath his premises as safe keeping for his customer's valuables, thus establishing the earliest safe deposit system. During the eighteenth and nineteenth centuries, vaults for valuables proliferated all over Britain as the country became more prosperous.

During World War II, underground space was commandeered for the storage of the treasures of Britain - those priceless objects of our long historical heritage without which Britain would be irreversibly spiritually impoverished. By the outbreak of war in 1939, the National Gallery had deposited

94

2000 of its most important paintings in provincial centres, but the subsequent blitz of several of those centres led to their trans-ference into a much more secure repository. This was the Manod Slate Mines, near Blaenau Ffestiniog in North Wales, where a series of brick galleries were hurriedly fashioned within the quarried chambers three hundred feet deep in the mountainside. Special air-conditioning plant was installed and the whole complex protected by large blast-proof steel gates.

Other treasurers were deposited below ground in other places. The type specimens of the botanical and zoological collections of the Natural History Museum - the irreplaceable specimens from which the species were originally described-disappeared under rock cover in the Carthouse Quarry at Godstone in Surrey. Many other long-forgotten crypts, tunnels and worked-out mines found a new use as temporary stores for the contents of museums, colleges and libraries.

In 1974, two vast underground ammunition stores were put up for sale. They were at Eastleys, near Corsham, and Monkton Farleigh near Bradford-on-Avon, both in Wiltshire. Converted from abandoned workings of the Bath Stone Mines during the war, the ammunition dumps were of astounding dimensions - over two million square feet in area, comprising many miles of tunnel, three miles of conveyor belt and ancillary services - enough space in all to house twenty buildings the size of London's Centre Point office block. The government had finally relinquished them in 1967, and in 1974 a farming combine purchased them, though what use they could be is mystifying.

Pitfalls

The word 'pitfall', meaning an unexpected drawback or hindrance, is common in the English language, but its origin is known to very few. Pits such as deneholes were sometimes used for a very specialized form of hunting - the pitfall.

Animals caught in the chase would be driven by hounds towards a special area where hedges and ditches were arranged as a trap which would funnel the game towards a pit, into which it would fall. The Anglo-Saxon *Colloquy of Archbishop Aelfric* mentions such a form of hunting in .connection with boars, which were then plentiful in England. The complex of ditches, banks and deneholes at Joyden's Wood in Bexley, Kent, is believed by some to be the remains of just such a hunting trap, though with the increasing rarity of large game and the invention of firearms, such methods of hunting became obsolete, and have survived only in the netting of wildfowl.

Ice Houses

Before the invention of refrigeration a century and a half ago, the only way to have ice during the summer was to collect it in the wintertime and to store it in specially-designed subterranean ice-houses. Even today at many stately homes one can find strange little buildings, sometimes dressed in fanciful garb as Egyptian or Classical temples, which on investigation turn out to be the entrances to ice-houses.

Ice-storage methods were perfected in ancient Rome, where, during the time of Seneca (4 B.C.E. - 65 C.E.) ice was sold in shops and by streetsellers during the summertime. Britain, however, had to wait until the time of King Charles II before ice storage was introduced by his gardener, the appropriately -named Mr Rose, who brought back the idea from France after a visit to Versailles.

The ice-house's efficiency depended upon excellent insulation. It had to be made so that the melting of the ice placed in it during the winter would be slowed down as much as possible by the exclusion of warm air. When over two-thirds of the pit was below ground, then insulation was almost perfect and ice could be stored indefinitely. The form of ice-houses depended on the whims of their designers: dome or globe-shaped;

circular; rectangular; bell-shaped or cylindrical. The most convenient shape was ovoid, with the narrow end of the 'egg' pointing downwards. Usually the ice-pit was lined with cavity walls of brick, and the entrance was oriented northwards, opening on a passage sealed by heavy doors to exclude warm air. Often the passage had a bend to reduce air circulation when the doors were opened for the removal of ice.

Chapter Six

Tunnels of Legend

During my travels in search of tunnels, I have often been assured by local informants that an underground tunnel runs from some prominent landmark such as the church or manor house to some other important site, often several miles distant. The persistence and universal spread of these tales indicate an ingrained belief in the mysterious, perhaps some deeper folk memory of a lost art. This phenomenon has been noted by several writers on underground passages, who usually have explained it as owing to misinterpretation or exaggeration of real short passages. In his remarkable book *Secret Hiding Places* Granville Squires discussed the legend. His explanation was that the tunnels are often only deep and wide drains, sewers or water conduits. As corroboration he offered the observation that such tunnels often run in the direction of rivers. Other less plausible theories for manor-church tunnels explain them as escape routes to the sanctuary of the church, but the theory is untenable owing to the amount of work required to make a tunnel which then in any case would not be secret.

The average length of a legendary tunnel is about two miles, and to build one of that length would be a major engineering operation, the like of which was not seen in Britain before the eighteenth century mine drainage channels. Squires claimed that the longest reputed tunnel he had come across was all of twenty-five miles long - longer than the longest rail tunnel in use today! The implausibility of the legend led him to

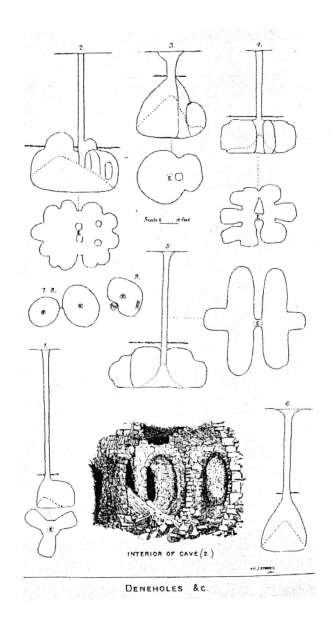

31. various patterns of southern English deneholes, as explored by F. C. J. Spurrell, 1881. (Nideck)

99

conclude that in the majority of cases the tunnels were completely imaginary.

If, as most people will agree, the majority of reputed tunnels are completely imaginary, how did the proliferation of such tales originate? The nineteenth-century expert on deneholes, F. C. J. Spurrell recounted an incident which may explain the origin of at least some of them:

> "Living as I did in a country where deep holes
> abounded, whose bottoms no one knew of, and whose
> intercommunication by endless passages over miles
> of country was the universal belief -lone useless and
> deserted in the depths of woods- it would have been
> strange indeed if I had not examined them with some
> care . . . As an instance of the origin of such legends, I
> once came across a man who told me that he had
> fallen down a pit, in which he passed two days. On
> recovering from the fall he wandered down deep
> passages for immense distances, until, regaining the
> entrance, he sat under it and howled until someone
> heard him (for a path led near the hole) and he was
> extricated."

Spurrell asked the man to show him the exact place where this happened, and subsequently explored the hole. But when he entered it 'no passages presented themselves; but the size of the cavern, its great circuit, its buttresses and pillars, and high irregular mounds of earth fallen from the vault, fully explained the account of the poor fellow, who, bruised, starved and in darkness, had crawled round and round the cave "in wandering mazes lost"

In his seminal work *The Old Straight Track*, published, in 1925, Alfred Watkins noted that legends of underground passages between ancient sites such as churches, abbeys, castles and camps are often on leys. Like many researches before and after, Watkins never verified one of these tunnels,

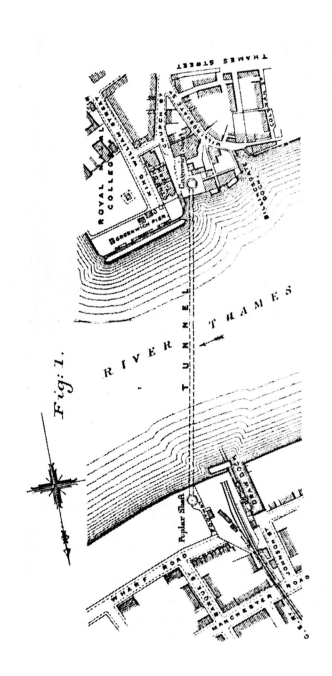

32. The River Thames at London was the first river to be tunnelled in modern times. This is a plan of the foot tunnel between the Isle of Dogs and Greenwich, now being paralleled by a new tunnel for the trains of the Docklands Light Railway (Electric Traction Publications)

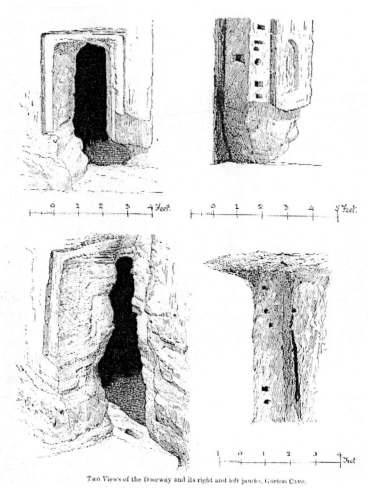

Two Views of the Doorway and its right and left jambs, Gorton Cave.

33. *Traditional human-made subterranea sometimes have architectural features, such as windows and doors. The cave at Gorton, in the valley of the Esk, south of Edinburgh, Scotland, is such a place. Drawing by F. R. Coles, 1897 (Nideck)*

but he would not discount the possibility of their existence. As the distance between many of the sites is impossibly long, and the terrain traversed is often rugged and difficult, Watkins believed that the legend was the folk memory of an old straight track along the alignment. He mentions the 1865 map of Hereford which marked a reputed tunnel linking the priory of St Guthlac with its vineyard on the banks of the River Wye. Several times the passage had fallen in or been dug into, and Watkins and a fellow member of the Woolhope Club excavated it. They found that it was no more than a natural fissure in the rocks.

One day near Llanthony Abbey, Watkins was using a sighting compass on a tripod in an attempt to locate a hill notch on the horizon. A passing workman halted and told him that local tradition told of an underground passage from that place to Llanthony. Watkins knew he was on an alignment to Llanthony, yet it was not visible because of the intervening ridge, so he concluded that the tunnel legend was a symbolic way of saying that a straight track traversed the ridge to an invisible point on the other side.

In *The Ley Hunter's Manual*, published in 1927, Watkins notes that when calling at Llangorse, Breconshire, he asked the postmaster, Mr Price, whether there were any legends about the nearby lake. Price replied 'Only that they always say there is an underground passage from Llangorse Church to Castle Dinas', a tunnel which would go straight through a mountain. Plotting this tunnel on his map, he found a ley, as such underground passages (which by this time he believed no-one had ever seen) 'are always on leys'.

In *The Ley Hunter* magazine No. 88, Paul and Jay Devereux describe just such a ley-tunnel. The Coldrum Ley in Kent, which runs from Trottiscliffe Church to Blue Bell Hill via the Coldrum stones, a crossways, Snodland church, an ancient ford on the River Medway and Burnham Court Church, incorporates a legendary tunnel, which, like those mentioned by Watkins, has never been found. The interesting point of this tunnel is that whilst all the other points on the ley are intervisible, the Coldrum Stones and Trottiscliffe Church are not - just as Watkins noted at Llanthony. A legend associated with the tunnel says that two brothers discovered it, and one decided to explore it whilst the other followed on the surface. The first brother entered, playing his flute, and, as is usual in the legends, the sound continued for some distance before suddenly ceasing. The surviving brother did not dare to enter to find out what had happened. The tunnel is also reputed to conceal treasure, which the authors believe may be a folk-memory of another geomantic site on the ley, now lost.

Paul Screeton, another writer on geomantic topics, notes the tunnel-ley relationship in his book *Quicksilver Heritage* in which a supposed tunnel on a ley in Teeside is mentioned. The ley has five points, running Billingham church - Norton Church - Redmarshall Church - Bishopton Castle Hill - Walworth Castle, and between Billingham and Norton is a reputed passage. However, the land between these churches is low-lying and prone to floods, making it impossible terrain for subterranea. The ley hypothesis is the only logical explanation.

Places linked by legendary tunnels are usually the prominent buildings of the neighbourhood: the parish church, the manor house, the main inn, a local abbey or nunnery, the castle, perhaps a mill, a prominent hill or outcrop of rock. In many districts where the geology of the terrain would make tunnelling easy, the legends are plausible. Indeed in towns such as Glastonbury and Nottingham at least some of the legendary tunnels have been verified by exploration. In most places, however, the terrain renders tunnels an impossibility. This is especially true of the tunnels which are said to burrow beneath rivers, for before the Thames Tunnel, built in the first half of the nineteenth century, tunnelling beneath rivers was impossible owing to the immediate flooding which ensues when a shaft or passage is cut through permeable rock below the level of the water table. That, after all, is the principle of the well. General tunnelling technique was to keep just above the water table. Some of the caves under Nottingham and the remarkable bell-shaped structure beneath the crossroads at Royston in Hertfordshire were so close to the average water table that in times of exceptional rainfall they still flood.

In towns with a monastic tradition, tunnel legends are invariably attached to the remains of the Abbey or Priory. In places where a nunnery existed relatively near to a monastery, tales of illicit meetings between monks and nuns are linked with the secret passageways. A classic example of the tale is found in Cambridge. Before the reformation there were two major monastic settlements to the east of the town, the Nunnery of St Radegund (now Jesus College) and Barnwell Priory. Both had associated holy wells, St Radegund's Well being now sealed and beneath the Rhadegund public house in King Street and the Bairns' Well (Barnwell) being lost under nineteenth century housing at Riverside. Between these two large and wealthy establishments, a tunnel is said to run. The length of the passage would be about three-quarters of a mile, cut through water-bearing gravel alongside the River Cam in ground which was frequently flooded. Its function, so legend asserts, was to facilitate love affairs between the inmates of the two establishments.

Of course, the passage is purely imaginary, for if the geology had permitted its construction, the Prior and Mother Superior would not have. If the legends are garbled folk-memories of some more esoteric link, however, we may be able to determine the nature of these links by observing other phenomena. Directly on the line of the supposed Radegund's-Barnwell tunnel is the Abbey House, a large old house built in part from the stones of the demolished Priory. There, over many years, psychical phenomena have plagued the residents. The phenomena have included a grey or white lady who has appeared on several occasions. She is naturally supposed to be the wraith of a nun who came by passage to meet her monastic lover, and who probably suffered some vile death for her transgressions. Other psychical activity at the Abbey House have included poltergeist phenomena which have torn off bedclothes.

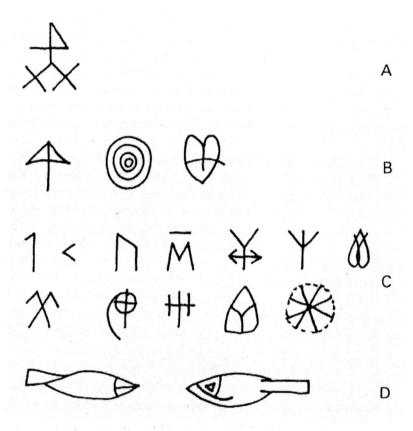

34. Symbols are found carved on the walls of many subterranea. These are a typical selection: (a) The Externsteine; (b) The Royston Cave; (c) the Burgstein; (d) Gloucester Cathedral Crypt. (Nigel Pennick)

The esoteric, geomantic or psychic explanations of long-distance tunnels cannot be discounted, as such legends, even on a much grander scale, are found throughout the world. In about 1844, a Peruvian priest who was summoned to absolve a dying Quechua Indian received a remarkable story about a system of underground tunnels beneath the Andes. The dying native told of the sealing of a secret tunnel-labyrinth by the High Priest of the Temple of the Sun under the aegis of the consort of the last Inca emperor Atahuallpa. Between 1848 and 1850 Helena Blavatsky visited Peru and was told of the tunnel, receiving a plan which is lodged in the Theosophical Archives at Adyar, Madras, India. 'We had in our possession an accurate plan of the tunnel, and the hidden, pivoted, rock-doors', wrote Madame Blavatsky, yet it has never been found.

Legends of massive tunnel systems running beneath the whole surface of the earth abound in esoteric publications. Often they are supposed to be ramifications of the legendary tunnel system connected with the subterranean city of Agharthi. According to Harold Wilkins in *The Mysteries of Ancient South America*, the South American continent is penetrated by a massive tunnel which is said to run from the Atacama Desert in Chile northwards into Peru linking various important Inca sites with the capital city, Lima. From that city, a branch of the tunnel, or *Socabon del Inca* is reputed to run all the way to the ancient Inca capital Cuzco. East of Cuzco, Wilkins's map shows a 'mysterious extension' through which the 40,000 refugees under the Inca resistance leader Tupa Amaru fled from Pizarro's *conquistadores* to a lost city in Brazil or northwest Bolivia.

A continuous tunnel over 900 miles long is obviously purely legendary, yet it may be a folk-memory of the geomantic system of holy lines which cover that country. In his book *Pathways to the Gods*, Tony Morrison describes the network of lines which connect *huacas* or holy places with perfect alignments akin to the leys of Alfred Watkins. The tunnel-ley connection noted by Watkins is certainly a strong possibility in Peru.

Tales of the supposed tunnel system continue to surface, having been dealt with in more recent time by Erich von Däniken and other proponents of the ancient astronaut theory. Wilkins believed that the tunnels were the remnants of Atlantean culture: the 'mysterious engineering of an antediluvian world'. This Atlantean connection of ancient tunnel legends is often linked with the mystical city of Agharthi. Esoteric tradition asserts that the Atlanteans, having by their offences against the natural order wiped out their homeland, migrated into Asia where they tunnelled beneath the Himalayas. There, esotericists believe, dwell to this day the mysterious 'White Brotherhood' or 'White Lodge' ruled by the King of the World, awaiting the time when again they shall emerge to rule this planet. The tradition is recounted in Ferdinand Ossendowski's *Beasts, Men and Gods* (1923). The Polish explorer and mystic claimed to have a prophecy uttered by the master of Agharthi, the so-called King of the World, who is supposed to have suddenly appeared at the Temple of Narabanchi, Outer Mongolia, in 1890.

The prophecy related to the coming half-century in which vast destruction and social upheaval would occur, followed by a period of peace, a further major war and then 'The peoples of Agharthi will come up from their subterranean caverns to the surface of the earth.'

It has been claimed that agents of the Nazi Occultist Heinrich Himmler attempted to reach Agharthi in order to enlist the assistance of the King of the World in their attempt at world domination. The connection between the legendary Agharthi and the Hell of the Judaeo Christian religions is not difficult to see. One of the titles traditionally appended to the Devil during the middle ages was *Rex Mundi* - King of the World.

Several writers have put Agharthi variously in Tibet, Outer Mongolia, the Hindu Kush or Afghanistan. Supposedly a land of peace, plenty and longevity, it was the model for Hollywood's Shangri-La, a name which echoes Shambhallah, another subterraneous city in the mould of Agharthi. The Tibetan connection is the most favoured, for the Potala at Lhasa, erstwhile seat of the Dalai Lama, supreme head of the Tibetan Buddhist church, was said to be connected directly with Agharthi by a system of tunnels like those in the Andes. Again, an esoteric or magical explanation is far more likely than a physical one. But it is not only Asia and South America which are supposed to be undermined by tunnels left over from the Atlantean Empire. In his curious work *Archaic England*, published in 1919, Harold Bayley tells of tunnels burrowed beneath much of Africa. One, said to pass beneath the River Kaoma, was supposed to be so long that it took his caravan from sunrise to noon to pass through it.

Even the prospect of tunnels hundreds of miles long has not been enough for some speculative writers. They have claimed that the whole planet Earth is not a solid ball of rock at all, but merely a sort of hollow sphere with access to the inhabited interior through vast holes situated at the poles.

In 1906, William Reed published *The Phantom of the Poles*, in which he claimed that 'the earth is not only hollow, but that all, or nearly all of the explorers have spent much of their time past the turning-point, and have had a look into the interior of the earth'. His belief was that at or near each pole there is a vast aperture, into which many polar explorers had inadvertently wandered. 'The poles so long sought are phantoms... in the interior are vast continents, oceans, mountains and rivers. Vegetable and animal life are evident in this new world, and it is probably peopled by races yet unknown to the dwellers upon the earth's exterior.'

Several explorers of the polar regions are supposed to have gone 'over the edge' and entered this inner world. The American Admiral Richard Byrd is said to have overflown both poles by over 1700 miles without returning to known territory, and tales of unknown forests inhabited by exotic fauna abound in connection with these unverifiable accounts. The speculative UFO researcher Brinsley Le Poer Trench claimed in *The Secret of the Ages: UFOs from inside the Earth* that unidentified flying objects might originate from an inner civilization which is plotting the overthrow of the upper world. Other weird phenomena like phantom animals and 'Fortean' happenings might also originate in the inner world, it was suggested.

Another proponent of the hollow earth-UFO connection is Roy Palmer, editor of the American UFO magazine *Flying Saucers*. Several deathbed accounts given by old sailors have been cited as evidence that the earth is indeed hollow, and the theme has proved interesting to writers of fiction. Palmer published the most noteworthy book in the genre, *The Smoky God* by Willis George Emerson, a tale of an old Norse sailor, Olaf Jansen, who sails over the top into the new world of the hollow Earth. But in reality, there is no evidence for the theory. Satellites and cosmonauts have been photographing the earth from space for over forty years, and the polar regions have been almost completely mapped on the ground and from aircraft.

Another supposed entrance to the subterranean kingdom was through the great whirpool known as the Maelstrom. Gerhard Kramer, better known as the cartographer Gerardus Mercator, placed this legendary abyss as a geographical location at the point where the four world ocean currents run into the Polar Gulf. It was believed at the time that the waters at that point descended thence into the underworld. The mystic seventeenth-century scientist Athanasius Kircher contended that a subterranean world was entered at the

Maelstrom whose waters came to the surface again at the Gulf of Bothnia, the northernmost part of the Baltic Sea between Sweden and Finland.

The use of the subterranean kingdom as a literary device has been widespread. Alice entered Lewis Carroll's Wonderland by falling down a shaft. The mystic users of the arcane force *vril* in Bulwer Lytton's influential novel *The Coming Race* resided in an underground land, which also was entered by a shaft accidentally discovered by a mine engineer at the end of an ancient tunnel. Such ideas may have been suggested by the tales of miners who occasionally do break into ancient workings such as those recently found during the construction of the Metro under Gateshead.

Yet another underground land appears in Jules Verne's *A Journey to the Centre of the Earth*, and the cannibalistic Morlocks of H. G. Wells's *The Time Machine* reside amid throbbing machinery in a vast network of tunnels connected to the surface by vertical shafts. That theme is taken up in many later science fiction works, where underground cities abound. The common features of the genre are found in the book *Etidorhpa, or The End of the Earth* by John Uri Lloyd, published in 1896. Here, the hero, Johannes Llewellyn Llongollyn Drury, son of a mythical occultist, is conducted through a subterranean kingdom. A strange alien being, bald and eyeless but of enormous strength, leads the hero into an - underworld where, after passing through the obligatory dark tunnel, he reaches a 'zone of inner light'. In this zone are the usual giant toadstools, pterodactyls and other monstrous reptiles; elsewhere other mysteries are shown to Drury as he is led from cavern to cavern.

This 'zone of inner light' is common to occult and literary accounts of the underground world. Often it is said to be a strange green glow which favours the growth of plant life. Such illumination is mentioned by Verne in *A Journey to the*

Centre of the Earth, Etidorhpa and even in the *Rupert The Bear* comic strip! Apart from being a convenient literary phenomenon, it has been reported by occultists as being the illumination of subterranean cities like Agharthi and Shambhallah. Apologists of ancient civilizations would attribute this to the lost sciences of Atlantis. Those with a more mystical inclination would cite the legendary Buddha sitting in a cave surrounded by his own illumination, and stories of initiates travelling to their esoteric masters in the astral body indicate a more supernatural explanation. But returning to the material world, we must dismiss these tales and rumours as mere myth: exaggerations of existing tunnels and rock-cut monasteries; garbled folk-memories of ancient troglodytic races; or representative of alternative realities on another plane of being. Whatever the truth, simple geographical exploration, mining and speleological research cannot help us unravel these mysteries.

Chapter Seven

Legends of the Subterranean World

To those who have not entered them, every hole in the ground, natural crevice and mine is a separate world of mystery, an enigmatic place where the reality of the world of light may be subtly altered by the forces of the earth and darkness. Gnomes, ogres, monsters and demons were universally reputed to reside in underground places and for mere mortals to enter them without some sort of physical and magical protection was held to be the height of folly. The many legends of lost explorers in tunnels attest to this idea.

The entrance to a tunnel or passage was seen as literally the entrance of the underworld, and as such had its guardian. In some legends, such as that of Ali Baba and the Forty Thieves or Child Rowland, the subterranean kingdom is entered through a magic door which only opens at the utterance of the appropriate password. Perhaps this is a garbled folk-memory of the entrances to the dwellings of troglodytes, who, wary of strangers, would only open their doors to friendly folk who knew their language. Sacred grottoes, too, would have had their guardians; the Cimmerians at the Grotto of the Oracle of the Dead at Baiae are a documented instance of this.

Even in modern times the tale of the door into the underworld is still as potent as ever. A story told by Helena Blavatsky's travelling companion Colonel Olcott is a modern version of

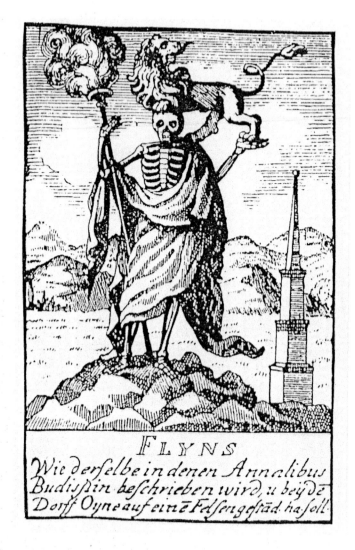

FLYNS
Wie derselbe in denen Annalibus Budißin beschrieben wird, u. beyde Dorff Oyne auf eine Felsengestäd ha soll.

35. *Traditionally, the underworld has its guardians and guides of the dead such as the Slavic god Flyns or Velin, shown here with his flaming staff that illuminates the underworld. An engraving from Samuel Grosser's work, Lausitzische Merkwürdigkeiten (Leipzig, 1714) (Nideck)*

the legend, in which the pair are supposed to have entered a rock-cut shrine in India in order to commune with the mystic Theosophical Masters. Olcott was engrossed in the commanding view from the cave's mouth when he noticed Blavatsky had disappeared. Suddenly there was sardonic laughter and the slamming of a heavy door, of which, however, there was no sign. Olcott searched the shrine, but there was nowhere she could have gone. Half an hour later, she suddenly appeared, having been through a secret door to converse with one of the hidden masters of Agharthi deep within the rock.

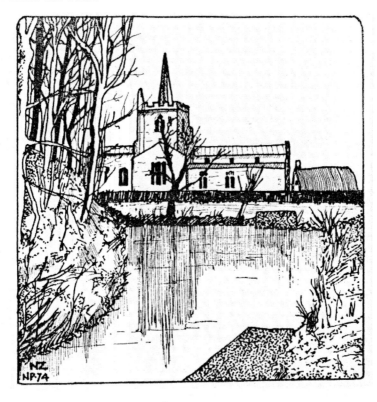

36. The church and moat at Anstey, Hertfordshire, England, where the Irpon gates were discovered. (Nigel Pennick)

Whether we accept this story at face value or dismiss it as fantasy, its symbolic content tallies exactly with other tales of the underworld. Unlike most penetrators of the subterranean kingdom, Helena Blavatsky returned unharmed. The entrances of caves and tunnels are more often than not seen as the mouth of the underworld - the gateway to Hell. A tunnel near Anstey in Hertfordshire, in which the legendary blind fiddler met his end, was reputed locally to be the mouth of Hell. His story enshrines all the major features of such legends, and is recounted later on. The place where the tunnel begins is now called Cave Gate, but before the Victorian sensibilities of the Ordnance Survey put this name on the map, it was known as Hell's Gate. Places like this were believed to be the literal site of an incident formerly commemorated in Christian sacred history but nowadays held to be apocryphal. In the *Gospel of Nicodemus* is a passage known commonly as the Harrowing of Hell in which Jesus Christ's spirit, during the period between the crucifixion and the resurrection, enters hell to liberate the souls of the just. In medieval iconography, the mouth of Hell is often portrayed as the mouth of a dog. Christ is shown holding open these jaws with his pastoral staff as Abraham and his flock emerge from the clutches of Satan. The whole episode is, of course, a story derived from the final labour of Hercules.

The Greek author Apollodorus gives the following account of this in his book *The Library:*

> A twelfth labour imposed on Hercules was to bring Cerberus from Hades. Now this Cerberus had three heads of dogs, the tail of a dragon, on his back the heads of all kinds of snake ... Having come to Taenarum in Laconia, where is the mouth of the descent to Hades, he descended through it. But when the souls saw him, they fled, save Meleager and the Gorgon Medusa. And Hercules drew his sword against the Gorgon, as if she were alive, but he learned from Hermes that she was an empty phantom. And being

come near the gates of Hades he found Theseus and Pirithous, him who wooed Persephone in wedlock and was therefore bound fast. And when they saw Hercules, they stretched out their hands as if they should be raised from the dead by his might. And Theseus, indeed, he took by the hand and raised up, but when he would have brought up Pirithous, the earth quaked and he let go.

A remarkable image of the Christian version of this legend can be seen in the stained glass windows of King's College Chapel in Cambridge, where a demon peers out of the monstrous maw of Hell. Other representations show Christ leading the souls of Noah, Abraham and other righteous people out from the clutches of Satan.

The Herculean legend incorporates the second major feature of the entry to the underworld, the guardian hound. The dog is, of course, primarily a guardian of entrances. The dog of Gwynn ap Nudd, Celtic god of the underworld and the faery kingdom, was named Dormarth, which means 'the gate of sorrow'. Gwynn's holy mountain, Glastonbury Tor, is eminently suited as a place of initiation for its sides are sculptured with a vast earthen labyrinth and local lore attests to the presence of several caves or tunnels cut into the rock of the holy hill. In the twelfth labour of Hercules, the hero had to bring out Cerberus from Hades, on condition that he was to use no weapons to accomplish the task. Hercules wrestled the dog-monster with his bare hands and brought it into the middleworld by strength alone.

In British folklore, a dog often accompanies the piper or fiddler who bravely enters an underground passage and is then lost. Other folktales tell of a dog that enters alone and emerges later from another tunnel several miles away. A typical example of this is told of the Cave O'Caerlauch in Galloway, Scotland, where, in John MacTaggart's *Scottish*

117

Gallovidian Encyclopaedia, published in 1824, is the following: 'Cave O'Caerlauch. Tradition says, that no human eye has ever beheld the back side, or farthest extremity of this cave; that a dog once went into its mouth and came out at the Door O'Cairnsmoor, a place nearly ten miles from it; and when the tyke did come out he was found to be sung, as if he had passed through some fire ordeal or other.' (The word *sung* in this passage is a dialect rendering of the word singed i.e. burnt.)

There are two important connections between the dog and the underworld. The first is a psychic link, for in many places a phantom dog, generally known by its East Anglian name of Black Shuck, appears. These ghostly figures haunt lanes, footpaths, roads, ancient trackways, bridges, crossroads, gateways and passages; in fact everywhere that there is movement. Subterranean passages are links downward to the underworld of the dead and so enter this category.

The second connection is the part which dogs appear to have played in religious rites of ancient times, as priest, gods and goddesses have been found portrayed in the company of dogs, so it is possible that they may have had a role in the rites of initiation traditionally conducted deep beneath the earth.

In the sixth book of the *Aeneid*, Virgil observes that the first things seen by his hero as the priestess conducted him towards the river of the underworld were several dogs. Diodorus Siculus notes that the rites of Isis were preceded by the presence of dogs, and Pletho in his commentary on the *Magical Oracles of Zoroaster* observes that at the initiation of neophytes the priests produced phantom dogs. According to Lewis Spence in *The Mysteries of Britain*, as the initiate entered the gloomy subterranean kingdom during his ordeal, the presence of dogs may have entered symbolically into the ceremony.

In the fiddler-dog legends, often the dog survives when the man does not. This may be a memory of the guardian dog which is friendly to souls entering the underworld but which prevents their re-emergence into the land of the living. Hence the struggle between the three-headed hound Cerberus and Hercules whilst leaving the netherworld. The cave or tunnel is envisaged as the aperture in the earth's surface through which the dead may travel to the nether- world, but with the possibility of rebirth. It is in this way that such passages were used in the various rites of initiation - if the postulant succeeded in overcoming the ordeals he was reborn into enlightment, but if he failed, then death ensued.

The Gundestrup Cauldron is an enigmatic silver vessel which was discovered in a Danish bog in 1891. A great deal of analysis, discussion and argument has been made over the cauldron, whose stylistic motifs are ambiguous, combining Thracian with Celtic symbols. One scene the meaning of which is still subject to argument, is of especial interest to students of the subterranean kingdom. In this scene, crested knights approach a sanctuary through a tunnel garlanded with leaves. Attended by a dog, a priest holds a child head downwards over a vessel or shafthead. In this position he appears to be about to make a human sacrifice. Much discussion over the meaning of the scene has taken place, but it is interesting to note that similar scenes may be witnessed in England today during the ceremony of Beating the Bounds. The ceremony is carried out by Church officials and laypersons during the period of Rogationtide, in order to reaffirm the boundary of the parish in which the ceremony is taking place. The people assemble at a traditional place on the boundary and start to walk along it, beating important geomantic markers such as stones, crosses and mark-trees as they pass them. At certain pre-arranged places, small cross-shaped trenches are cut in the ground and a child is picked up by the legs and placed head-first in the hole. Stones are cast into the hole, which is then filled in.

This ritual is possibly the memory of a human sacrifice made when the boundary was originally laid out. The similarity with the image on the Gundestrup Cauldron is striking. The casting of objects into special ritual shafts was relatively commonplace and such shafts have been excavated at Long Wittenham in Buckinghamshire and at Holzhausen, Bavaria. Sometimes a whole tree would be cast into the hole, and the Gundestrup Cauldron shows this. Until the last century, the standard means of blocking abandoned deneholes and chalk wells was by throwing down whole trees and then infilling with agricultural rubbish.

Ritual shafts were not only access points to the underworld, but also markers in the ancient survey of the country. The antiquary Sir Montagu Sharpe, whose excellent work on the Roman survey of Middlesex is all but forgotten today, showed that at important points on the survey, the *agrimensores* dug shafts known as *arcae* which acted as geodetic markers. The position of the Royston Cave, which is dealt with in detail below, is just such a place.

The entrance to the subterraneous world needs a guardian only if there are people brave or foolhardy enough to penetrate it. British folklore seems to put local musicians in this category, for it is usual to find a piper, fiddler or drummer being egged on by his friends and neighbours to brave the uncertain dangers of an unexplored tunnel.

In England, the explorer is rarely a piper, for bagpipes only survived as a folk instrument in Northumbria, Scotland and Ireland. The English caver is usually a fiddler, sometimes blind. The typical feature of this legend has been recounted already in the Coldrum Ley, and it exists at Anstey in Hertfordshire, where a passage exists today in the side of a chalk-pit. The passage, which begins at Cave Gate, is said to run eastwards for a mile to the castle at Anstey where it emerges through iron gates into the moat. Like the legendary tunnels at Binham Priory in Norfolk and Grantchester Manor near Cambridge, a fiddler entered never to return.

The story of the Anstey tunnel is as follows. One evening in early autumn, the day's work being finished, the farm labourers were drinking at the Chequers Inn, enjoying the music of the fiddler, Blind George. The labourers' conversation turned to the subject of the cave, and most agreed that it was a place to be avoided by anyone who was not a saint. Blind George threw down his fiddle on the bench in anger at this, and swore that, blind as he was, and accompanied by only his dog and fiddle, he would venture that very night to the utmost end of the passage. Everybody left the Chequers and walked to the pit to witness this feat of bravery. Dragging his reluctant whining dog with him, Blind George entered the cave playing. The Chequers regulars followed the music along the surface, and they had travelled about half the distance to Anstey Castle when the fiddling suddenly stopped. A horrific shriek was heard, followed by stony silence.

The throng rushed back to the entrance as fast as it could, but there was nothing to be seen, and none dared enter. After a while, a frantic scuffling was heard, and the now tailless dog suddenly appeared with all its hair burnt off. When it saw the crowd, it scrambled up the opposite side of the pit with a howl, and ran off never to be seen again. The villagers had had enough of these sinister happenings and fled to their homes. Early the next morning, they went to the cave to look for Blind George, but there was no sign, so they decided to wall up the entrance with flint rubble and mortar.

The tale is purely legendary, as the tunnel was explored in 1965 and found to go only a few yards. Anstey church registers show that at the end of the seventeenth century there was indeed a fiddler named George, but he lies in the churchyard, not the cave.

In Scotland, it is a piper who braves the unknown. The legend is typified by that of the Piper's Cave O'Gowend in Galloway, recorded in 1800 by the Parish Minister A. MacCulloch, and re- counted in the *Statistical Account* published at Wigtown in 1841: 'Coves or Caves. There are a number of these on the "wild shores of caverned Colvend"'. The principal of these is called the Piper's Cove, from a legend that a piper undertook to explore it. He carried his pipes with him, and continued to play underground till he reached Barnbarrach, about four miles distant from its mouth. The sound then ceased, and nothing was ever heard again of the unfortunate minstrel. It is found, however, to be only a hundred and twenty yards in length.'

John MacTaggart described the same cave in the *Scottish Gallovidian Encyclopaedia*. 'It is situated on a lonely shore, and frequently is heard the sound of bagpipes therein; some think the piper a devil, others fancy the musician to be some kind ofcarline (ghost - N.P.), who reveres the memory of departed highlanders, who were anciently smothered in the cave.'

At Dunskey Castle, near Portpatrick in Galloway, Waiter de Curry, who lived there in the fourteenth century, was accustomed to carry out acts of piracy on the Irish coast. He brought back from one foray a captive Irish piper whom he forced to serve as his personal musician. The piper's sense of humour was too abrasive for his master's liking, and the hapless musician was consigned to a dungeon to die. The piper found a secret passage leading from the dungeon, but became trapped in it and starved to death. Subsequently, his ghost has been heard along the line of the supposed tunnel piping as he was accustomed to do in life.

When workmen were constructing the Portpatrick water supply and drainage system in about 1900, they 'stumbled upon a large cavernous space as the very place where the reputed sounds of the ghostly pipe music were heard'. (J. Maxwell Wood, *Witchcraft and Superstitious Record in the South- Western District of Scotland, 1911*.) The legend current in the 1970s had the tunnel running almost a mile from the castle to the District Nurse's house at Portpatrick Harbour.

It has often been suggested that the Scottish piper legends might be derived from the weird sounds caused by the tides compressing air in caves. The air is then forced to escape through fissures in the rock, making ghostly wailing noises. This phenomenon can be observed near coastal caves, but the similarity of the stories with those of drummers or fiddlers eliminates the phenomenon as the sole origin of the legends.

The motive behind the musicians' entry to the tunnels seems to have been bravado or curiosity. However, the lure of buried treasure is also a strong motivation. Treasure legends of the underworld usually involve supernatural guardians, often those animals associated with witchcraft and death. One such legend, from Leeds, incorporates almost everything. An old man was working one day in the meadows surrounding the ruins of Kirkstall Abbey on the outskirts of the city. During his midday meal break, he went for a walk and came across a hole he had never seen before. On entering the hole, he found a tunnel which led to a great underground room with a huge fire blazing on the hearth. In one corner stood a black horse, behind which was a large wooden chest upon which sat a black cock. The labourer strode across the room to the chest and lifted the lid, whereupon an owl screeched and an unseen club descended across his head. When he regained conscious-ness, he was lying on the grass by the abbey, and nobody could ever find the hole again.

Clearly, the hole was more than a mere tunnel: it was an access point into a separate dimension or reality. Another supernatural access point was at the Craig Y Ddinas cave near Glynedd in Wales. Here it is said that a wizard once came upon a Welsh drover carrying a hazelwood staff and asked him to take him to the tree from which the staff had been cut. When they reached the tree, the wizard uprooted it and revealed a tunnel leading to the cave, at the entrance of which they discovered a bell. In the gloom the drover and wizard could just discern the outlines of King Arthur and his knights sleeping by a vast pile of silver and gold. The wizard instructed the drover to take as much of the treasure as he wanted, but never to touch the bell; but accidentally touching the bell, the drover woke the knights, who asked, 'Is it the day?' The drover replied with the stock answer,'No, sleep on.' A second accidental ringing again woke the knights, who were quelled by the same reply. The third time he touched the bell, he forgot to answer and was so badly beaten that he was crippled for life.

A similar King Arthur story is told at Richmond in Yorkshire, where a potter named Thompson is reputed to have found a secret tunnel which ran beneath the castle. Following it, he came to a deep cavern where King Arthur and his knights lay sleeping. By them lay a horn and a sword. Potter Thompson picked up the horn and was about to blow it when the knights began to stir. Terrified, he fled, and as he did so, he heard a voice say 'Potter Thompson, Potter Thompson, if thou hadst drawn the sword or blown the horn, Thou hadst been the luckiest man ever born.' This passage is unique in being the site of the two common tunnel legends for it is also related locally that a drummer boy was once sent along the tunnel to see whether it led to Easby Abbey one and a half miles away. His fellow soldiers, as in all such tales, followed the drumming along the surface, but about halfway it stopped. It is said that at certain times a ghostly drumming can be heard.

Torbarrow Hill at Cirencester has another living dead legend in which two men once discovered a chamber of a tunnel carved into the hillside. Entering the chamber they saw a knight who feebly struck out at their candle. Nearby, their attention was momentarily drawn to two perfectly-preserved embalmed bodies when the knight struck out again and extinguished their flame. A sudden moan in the darkness terrified the explorers who fled blindly to the exit whilst the cave collapsed behind them, sealing it forever.

Perhaps such legends are derived from illicit penetrators of burial vaults, who in search of grave gods, were disturbed by some guardian and put to flight only to ascribe supernatural agency to their eviction. Whilst the stories of human entrants to the underworld are commonplace, with variations on a theme of music or Arthurian guards, tales concerning animals are usually much more straightforward. Many places tell of dogs down some hole only to emerge at an unimaginably distant site.

A strange collection of fertility, animal and resurrection tales is attached to Palmer's Hole at Orleton Hill in Herefordshire. From the hole a twelve-foot long passage leads back to the surface. Until about a century ago, local youths would crawl through the short passage, as it was said that those who turned back or got stuck would never marry. A goose was once put down the hole, but it did not emerge via the twelve-foot passage. Instead, it was found some time later at Gauset, four miles away. The name Gauset is thus said to come from the exclamation 'Goose out!' called when it emerged from the other end of the tunnel. The Orleton hole also seems to be connected with a residue of *omphalos* lore, for it was believed that Orleton churchyard was the place where, on the morning of the Last Judgement, the dead would be first resurrected.

Animals put down tunnels seem to have fared more favourably than humans, who never usually re-emerged. But we are never told in the explorer myths what actually caused the untimely deaths of the brave explorers. Although treasure legends cite guardians, sometimes, as at Guiseborough Priory in Yorkshire, an animal which transforms itself into the Devil, in the musician tales there is not a trace of the agent. Presumably such things are hidden from mere mortals.

Demons

The subterranean kingdom seems to have a plethora of demonic denizens. On the Isle of Man, cave-noises are said to be made by the breathing of a sea-monster called the Cughtage, whilst on Enhgland, in the Danes Hills near Leicester was Black Annis's Bower. This was a fearsome cave where dwelt the eponymous demoness. Her activity was hunting little children, whom she devoured, and hung up their skins to dry at the cave's mouth.

Medieval Irish literature contains a series of stories called Caves, but few have survived intact. Two Irish caves, however, have a considerable body of legends attached to them, they are the Cave of Cruachan at Rathcroghan in County Roscommon, and St Patrick's Purgatory in County Donegal. The Cave of Cruachan, also called Ireland's Gate of Hell, was seen as a portal linking this world and the otherworld. It was greatly feared, as it was reputed to be the home of demons, and the source of plagues, "the fit abode" of the horrid Morrigan. At the festival of Samhain (hallowe'en), in t-Ellen trechend, 'the Three-Headed Ellen', and other demonic beings would come forth onto the Earth.These monsters included a destructive swarm of red-ochre coloured birds, 'The birds of the dead', whose breath withered fields and orchards. They were accompanied by a teeming throng of abominable otherworldly swine.

The belief that ogres, demons or giants inhabit the subterranean kingdom is very ancient. From the archaic myth makers to modern story-tellers like H. P. Lovecraft, tales of atrocities performed by demonic yet human troglodytes have fascinated their audiences. Ogres abound in folk tale, ranging from the utterly fantastic to the plausible. The more human legends include that of Sweeney Todd, the 'demon barber' of

Fleet Street with his murder cellar beneath the barber's chair and adjacent cannibal pie shop linked by an underground passage, and the tale of the Scottish troglodyte Sawney Beane and his horrific family.

The very existence of Sawney Beane has been hotly disputed. Some scholars see him as an ancient myth transplanted to the seventeenth century, whilst others believe his story to be based on fact. The legend describes him as a bandit whose penchant for human flesh led him to waylay and murder hundreds of luckless travellers crossing the trackless wastes of wild Galloway. His exploits and final capture and execution were first published at the end of the seventeenth century, portraying his as having lived about a century earlier. *The Legend of Sawney Beane* first appeared in about 1700 as a broadsheet typical of the popular press of the time. Broadsheets carried numerous subjects of popular interest, not the least of which were the activities of famous bandits, pirates, highwaymen and murderers. Of these many miscreants, only the names of Captain Morgan, Dick Turpin and Sawney Beane are still well known today.

Beane and his clan were reputed to inhabit a cave in Galloway, a remote part of Scotland noted for its wildness and barbarous inhabitants. In that part of the country there are many natural caves or 'coves', most of which have been cut in sea-cliffs over the ages by the action of the waves. The piper legends of Galloway have already been mentioned, and their caves are mostly named after famous local pirates or smugglers like Dirk Haterick. The broadsheets, however, refer to Beane's cavern as being a long passage 'which reached almost a mile underground'. This would rule out both a wave-cut coastal cave and also a man-made tunnel, for such lengths were not excavated before the mine drainage *soughs* of eighteenth century Derbyshire.

The connection between cannibalism, Beane's banditry and subterranea appears to be a folk memory of ancient troglodyte life. Cannibalism in ancient times was commonplace both in ritual and as a source of protein. The Beaker Folk, who lived in Britain about 4000 years ago, are known to have practised cannibalism from remains found in a refuse pit at Mildenhall Fen in Cambridgeshire which contained refuse of human bones suggestive of a cannibal feast. Even as late as 100 B.C.E., such practices were still in vogue. An Iron Age settlement at Danebury Hill in Hampshire has produced the remains of human bodies, mixed with the rubbish and bones of animals, and the troglodyte cannibals of Highfield Pits have already been noted. Tales of blood-crazed troglodytes may well be derived from these unpleasant people.

The possibility that the subterranean cannibals of antiquity were the remnants of an earlier race may also account for these legends. It has been suggested that when Celtic invaders arrived from Continental Europe in about 500 B.C.E., they drove the indigenous inhabitants into remote parts of the British Isles where they survived for many centuries as mysterious shadowy figures. They were small and of darker complexion than the Celts; they lived in caves or earth houses and were cannibals, at least for some of the time. It has been said that these earlier folk were the origin of the fairy and ogre legends which abound in these isles. Supporting evidence for this theory comes from the history of the Picts, a race which finally succumbed to genocide during the middle of the first millenium C.E. Archaeologists working on their dwelling-sites have shown that the Picts originally resided in underground earth houses, but at a specific period went over to building their drystone-walled defensive towers known as *brochs*.

An invading race finding the indigenous inhabitants living under ground in earth houses would see them as some sort of inferior beings, especially if their racial characteristics varied markedly from their own. The small size of many subterranean passages in earth houses attests to the smallness of the inhabitants, and may have helped promote ideas about gnomes in the subterranean kingdom. The dwarfs of Nordic mythology lived in a subterraneous world ruled over by their own king, Alberich. They only emerged from their tunnels at night, for to do so during the daytime was to be turned to stone. They were miners and craftsmen who worked metals, and naturally guarded secret knowledge of subterranean treasure, perhaps the whereabouts of metalliferous seams.

These points fall into perspective when we consider the theory of a conquered race. Living in subterranea, they would only emerge at night for fear of the new master race. Their secret knowledge might be astronomical, for they could have been the builders of the megalithic observatories appropriated by the Celtic Druids. Their treasure and skill in metal working is evidenced by the sumptuous grave goods found in pre-Celtic burials.

The smallness of the people who built the earth houses of Scotland and Ulster has long been a source of comment. James Farrer, who visited an earth house on the islet known as the Helm of Eday, Orkney, in 1855, remarked 'Whilst the size of the stones used in its construction is evidence of great personal strength on the part of the builders, the small and narrow rooms seem to indicate a diminutive race.' Another antiquary, J. R. Tudor, asked, 'What size could the people have been who crawled in through such rabbit holes as the passage of their eirde house are?' (*The Orkneys and Shetland, 1883*). In *An Account of Some Souterraizs in Ulster* read at the British Association meeting at Leicester in 1907, an Ulster archaeologist, Mary Hobson, said: 'The entrances are small, but the tiny doorways between one chamber and another are of even more diminutive dimensions - great numbers being too small to admit the average-sized man - a person having to

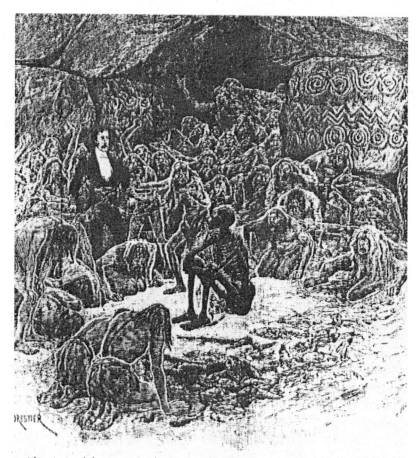

The grinning skeleton turned its head and regarded Rudolph from its eyeless orbs with a vacant glance of hungry satisfaction.

37. *A nineteenth century fantasy of the spectral denizens of ancient burial-mounds assaulting a Victorian gentleman. Engraving by A. Forestier, from* Pallinghurst Barrow *by Grant Allen, The Illustrated London News, Christmas edition, 1892. (Nideck)*

lie down flat in order to get through, and even then the width will not allow other than the shoulders of a woman or boy to pass through.'

It is obvious that nobody would construct buildings which they could not enter, so we must assume that the proportions of the builders were commensurate with the dimensions. Numerous remains of human habitation have been found in such subterranea, so the suggestion that they might have been made as spirit receptacles does not ring true.

It appears that the old race of inhabitants of Scotland and Ulster was comparable with the modern Eskimos in character and physical stature. The anthropologist Charles H. Chambers, writing in 1864 in the *Anthropological Review* said 'I believe the race which inhabited the northern shores of Europe to have been akin to the Lapps, Fins and Esquimaux, and the Pickts or Pechts of Scotland, and to have given rise to many of the dwarf, troll and fairy stories extant among the Sagas and elsewhere.' The year before this statement was made a discovery of twenty-seven human skulls in the island of Burray, Orkney was reported in *The Prehistoric Annals of Scotland*. They were 'of the Esquimaux type, short and broad'. Later we will see how the Eskimos (Innuit) actually inhabited similar earth houses, so it is possible that the peoples were identical.

Tales of underground gnomes and dwarfs are quite separate from other legends of the underworld, which are set in a mythological other world quite removed from the mundane earth-houses. For example, the Greek underworld had a complex and hierarchical structure, being divided into two areas: Erebus, where the souls of the dead were sent to wait; and Tartarus, a deeper and more impenetrable part. Various rivers divided the zones of Hades from the world of the living. First was Acheron, across which Charon the boatman ferried the souls of the departed for a fee - the coin traditionally left in the mouth or on the eyes of the corpse. If they could not pay the ferryman, then the souls were lost, and remained for ever in limbo on the banks of Acheron. Other rivers of the underworld were the river of forgetfulness Lethe; the famous Styx, by which the gods swore oaths of terrible power; Cocytus, the river of groans; and Phlegethon, the river of fire. Once in Hades, souls were judged by three magistrates; the damned were dispatched lower to Tartarus and the saved went to the paradise of the Elysian Fields.

This structure is very close to the Christian exegesis of the structure of Hell, and like the early Christian conception of Hell, which derived from it, Hades was penetrable by the living, and such concepts have survived in British folk-myths. The descent of Orpheus, Hercules and Jesus into the underworld to rescue loved ones or the righteous from the clutches of evil are echoed in an old Scottish folk-tale, *The Legend of Childe Rowland*. The earliest version of this tale is dated at around 1770, but it is certainly much older as part of it appears in the ravings of Edgar in Shakespeare's *King Lear* which was published in 1604. As it stands, it incorporates all the salient features of such myths.

A king had four children, a daughter Burd Ellen and three sons, the youngest of whom was Childe Rowland. Whilst playing ball on the roof, it was thrown off and Ellen was sent to get it back. When she did not return, each son in turn was sent to look for her, and finally, when two of the sons had also been lost, the youngest, Childe Rowland was dispatched. She had been captured by the King of Elfland, and was held prisoner inside a green mound. Childe Rowland walked round it thrice widdershins, then called 'Open door!' at which a dark cavern miraculously opened. Entering, he made his way to the Hall of the Elf King only to find his sister alive but his brothers dead. Tired by his long journey, he asked his sister for food, and, being under the influence of the ElfKing, she brought it. Just as he was about to eat it Rowland remembered that to eat in the underworld is to become trapped there, and threw the food to the ground. Magic having failed, the King himself rushed in bearing arms, crying:

With Fie and Foe and Fum,
I smell the blood of a Christian man,
Be he dead, be he living, with my brand,
I'll dash out his harns (brains) frae his harn-pan.

They fought, and Rowland overcame the demonic king who agreed to release Burd Ellen and restore Rowland's brothers to life. This done, Rowland spared the king, and the four left the Elf Kingdom and returned home in safety.

Although the legends of the underworld are complex and mysterious, they enshrine certain historical facts. The origin of some legends may rest in folk-memories of a former age, whilst others are derived from shamanistic experiences on the psychic planes. Yet other legends may have as their origin glimpses of actual rites practised below ground. Those of the German *Vehmgericht* have already been mentioned, the Oracles at Avernus and Baiae and the Mysteries of Eleusis are well-documented, for the use of subterranea in initiatory rites has several advantages. In all initiations, the ordeal factor is strong, and we find this in tunnel legends. Nowadays, the last remnant of the subterranean terrors of the neophyte is the fairground ghost train. Most magical societies nowadays cannot afford the luxury of hypogeal initiatory chambers; like the modern Freemasons, they find the use of the blindfold an acceptable subsititute.

As places of initiation, hypogea must have been places of sacred power. This power may either have occurred there naturally, or may have been specially generated by geomantic and magical acts. The sacred caves of oracles, such as that of Ramahavaly in Madagascar were examples of centres of natural power, whilst grottoes of the Virgin Mary such as that at Lourdes seem to have acquired power by supernatural means. By religious observances and pious feelings, the power in these subterranea have been contained and magnified, as evidenced by the numerous cures which still occur daily at Lourdes.

Like all energies, the power residing in such places can be channelled for either good or evil purposes. The benevolent energies of the Virgin are countered by the sinister machinations of the demonic empire. According to the *Book of Enoch*, St Michael's victory over the Devil resulted in the fallen angels being banished underground. Paracelsus believed that the abode of the demonic empire was below the earth, and various psychic manifestations are associated with subterranea old and new. Modern research on the relationship between psychical manifestations and earth energies indicates that sound may play an important part in the generation or dispersal of these phenomena, and indeed we find a specific correlation between sound and the legends of the subterranean kingdom. Traditionally, the explorers of tunnels are musicians who play as they walk; Arthur's knights are woken by a bell; the Pied Piper charms first the rats, then the children of Hamelin away to the subterranean kingdom with his pipe. And it was a universal superstition not to whistle in mines lest the Knockers should be provoked and cause a roof fall or explosion.

The suppression of the demonic empire by means of sound is well documented. Gongs, rattles, whistles, bells, fireworks, mantras, chants and hymns have been used in various parts of the world to suppress demonic interference during sacred rituals. The saints of the ancient Celtic church used to carry hand bells with them wherever they went in order to provide a correct psychic environment for their activities, and to exorcise the demons of the underworld from their monastic subterranea. The sound of fiddlers, drummers and pipers would also suppress the effectiveness of demonic spirits or

134

earth energies resident in the tunnels under exploration. Whatever the origins of these legends, the tunnels and subterranea which give rise to them will always be interesting in their own right. In the next chapter we will encounter the more enigmatic of the British subterranea-fogous, earth houses and deneholes.

Chapter Eight

Fogous, Earth Houses and Deneholes

The majority of subterranea found in Britain are of well-known types: the ice-houses, crypts, cellars, wells, mines, etc., which have well-defined structures and functions. Others like the Royston Cave are unique. But there are also three classes of structure whose origins and uses are enigmatic and which have given rise to many speculations and 'explanations'. They are the Fogous of Cornwall, the Earth Houses of Scotland and Ulster, and those mysterious shafts in the chalk known collectively as Deneholes.

Fogous

In Cornwall are to be found certain underground structures known by their Cornish name of Fogous. Their structure and plan are similar to the various underground buildings encountered in Scotland, Ireland, Scandinavia, Iceland, Shetland, the Orkneys and France. The name is derived from the word meaning 'cave', for in the Celtic group of languages the words *fougou, vouga, voo, vau, foe, ogo, oogo, hugo* and *googoo* have that meaning.

The Cornish antiquary William Borlase derived the name from *fo*, a place, and *govea*, to lie hidden, and calls them 'hiding places, dens or caves'. R. Williams, in his *Lexicon Cornu-Britannicum* (1865) translates *fo* as a retreat and *gow* as false or hidden, thus the word Fogou means a hidden refuge, an underground structure disguised so as to mislead a potential enemy, and indeed the features of known Fogous fit the bill.

Fogous are generally subterranean, being roofed with a series of large lintel stones resting on dry stone walling of a character in keeping with the Cornish 'hedges' or stone walls which divide the fields. Fogous have usually more than one entrance, opening on a main gallery. In addition there are often smaller side entrances (known as 'creeps') which are accessible only in the crawling position. Most Fogous consist of a curving gallery, which is sometimes oriented north-east to south-west. Construction was by making a trench, lining it with stone, then roofing it over with megalithic lintel-stones, the technique now called cut-and-cover and used in the construction of underground railways today. The entrances at each end provide access to the interior, and the whole Fogou is usually covered with an earth mound - a similar form of construction to the megalithic passage-graves of Eire. Sometimes, a Fogou may be completely embedded in a 'great wall'. These 'great walls', some of which reach twelve feet in thickness, are mysterious structures which have never been properly investigated. Their irregular shapes and great thickness render them inefficient as boundaries of fields and subterranean mysteries must lie undisturbed at the core of many of them.

The function of Fogous has long been a matter of contention. They never occur in isolation, being always an integral part of a settlement or fort in a stragetic position. Few artifacts have been discovered inside Fogous, and indeed very little which indicates their use as a dwelling of any kind. A typical Fogou is that at Pendeen Vau. Situated partly in a 'great wall', it was in the vicinity of Borlase's ancestral home at Pendeen Manor Farm. Henderson, in his *Mss. Antiquities*, quotes Borlase: 'It consists of three caves or galleries; the entrance is four feet six inches in high and as many wide, walled on each side with large stones, with a wide arch on the top . . . The sides built up of stone draw nearer together as they rise - the better to receive the flat stones which form the coverings, and are six feet from the ground. The first cave is twenty-eight feet long.'

Borlase noted the tiny creep, a 'square hole, two feet wide and two feet six inches high, through which you creep into the third cave, six feet wide and six feet high . . .' and attempted to find out the whole structure's function. 'I caus'd the floor of this Cave to be dug in two places, but found neither Cell nor Grave, but the natural ground only without any appearance of its having been mov'd.' He had no idea of what it was for, but recent discoveries and observations have shed more light upon these strange passages. The Fogou at Carn Euny in the parish of Sancreed is perhaps one of the best known, containing several unusual features which until recently were puzzling to antiquaries. Situated on a hillside which overlooks the southern and western coasts of Cornwall, the Fogou abuts on the remains of human habitation and a bronze age passage grave. At some time during the medieval period it was deliberately filled in like the oracular caves at Baiae. Near to the Fogou is a holy well dedicated to St Euny, an Irish saint who arrived with a party of colonists at the end of the fifth century. The observance of this saint's festival at Redruth was on Candlemas, so we must speculate that some Pagan tradition is associated with his sites.

The Fogou was excavated by Copeland Borlase in 1863-64, but today the Fogou is ruined, consisting of a stone-lined passage which has lost its roof. After about twenty-six feet, the roof is still intact, and forms a curving covered passage with thirty-three feet of tunnel, six feet high by six feet eight inches wide at the bottom. The total length of passages is sixty-six feet, and near the western end the customary creep leads to the surface. Both main entrances are oriented east-west. On the north side of the passage is a doorway which leads by way of a short passage to a circular chamber, now roofless, which archaeologists believe was never roofed with corbelled stone but was finished with some sort of timber and turf construction.

Sylvia Harris has drawn attention to an exciting mythological connection between the Carn Euny Fogou and Arthurian romance. In various versions of the Tristan and Isolde romance - the *Tristan* of Gottfried von Strassburg (c. 1210), the Norwegian *Tristramssaga* (1226) and the English *Sir Tristram* (late thirteenth century), there is a reference to a Cornish cave in which the lovers took refuge during their flight from the Court of King Mark. Gottfried von Strassburg claimed to have 'known since he was eleven' the location of the mysterious cave of the romance. In the tale, the place was described as a secret place in a hillside beside a certain water. It was vaulted and dug deep in the ground, which rules out a natural cave, and was protected by a holy tree. The ensemble is typical of the shrines created by the geomants of ancient Britain, combining natural and man-made features designed to emphasize and express the natural telluric energies of the place.

In yet another Tristan romance, that of the Anglo-Norman poet known only as Thomas, this underground structure is identified as a *locus amoenus* or Earthly Paradise, constructed in former times by giants. The form and dimensions of this unique place as depicted in the romances are virtually identical with those of the Carn Euny Fogou, and the holy well of St Euny was known locally as the Giant's Well until publication of the Ordnance Survey map gave it an official name.

The connection of ancient pagan religion with Fogous is apparent at Boleigh, where the Fogou contains an unique carving of a male figure. Discovered as late as 1957 by Dr E. B. Ford, the carving consists of a bas-relief two feet nine

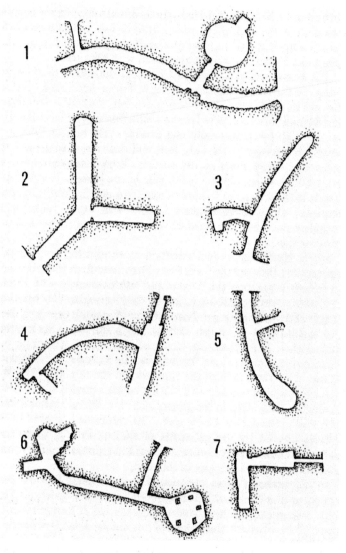

38. *Plans of typical Cornish Fogous, Scottish earth houses and Irish souterrains: 1. Carn Euny Fogou; 2. Pendeen Vau Fogou; 3. Boleigh Fogou; 4. Halligey Fogou, Trewarren; 5. Crichton earth house; 6. Saverock earth house, Kirkwall; 7. Ballyanly souterrain, Co. Cork, Eire.*

inches in height within a shield-shaped surround. The archaeologist C. A. Raleigh Radford believed that the carving was of the Romano-British or even the pre-Roman Celtic period. It represents a long-haired male grasping a spear in his upraised right hand, his left hand grasping a diamond-shaped object which has been interpreted as the head of a serpent which coiled about the spearman's wrist.

The famous effigy of the horned god on the Gundestrup Cauldron has such a snake-grasping hand, so this may be an attribute of a now-forgotten Celtic god. The condition of the stone at Boleigh suggests that it was not carved *in situ* in the Fogou, but brought from another place where it had already suffered weathering. This points to the stone being a sacred object from another site, incorporated in the Fogou as a sanctifier, which indicates a possible sacred use for Fogous in general. The carving on the stone, brought from another site, may represent the deity to whom the use of the Fogou was dedicated. The mysterious nature of such tunnels, with their complicated creeps and stumbling entrances, seems perfectly suited to the performance of strange rituals of the ancient mysteries. Whatever their uses, which certainly have not been determined to everybody's satisfaction, the Fogous remain without parallel in England. The *souterrains* of Ireland and the earth houses of Scotland, however, many of which were certainly used as dwellings, are sometimes of such similarity to the Fogous that some connection must be inferred.

Earth Houses

The term 'earth house' denotes an underground structure almost invariably built of stone and used primarily as habitation. In lowland Scotland, the terms *yird-hoose* or *eird-hoose* are applied to them, which corresponds with the Norse description *iord-hus*. In Gaelic they are known as *uamh*, pronounced *weem* by non-Gaelic speakers.

Earth houses have several well-defined characteristics. Their entrances are invariably narrow and often contain stumbling blocks to catch intruders. The best examples of stumbling blocks are found in Ireland, and are admirably demonstrated by the earth house at Rathmullen in County Down. Although this earth house is 120 feet long and generally six feet in height, the entrances at the barriers are a meagre two feet six inches high. These barriers are in some cases built from the floor upwards, but in other cases from the ceiling downwards as well. They are an integral part of the structure and their purpose is obviously to impede intruders.

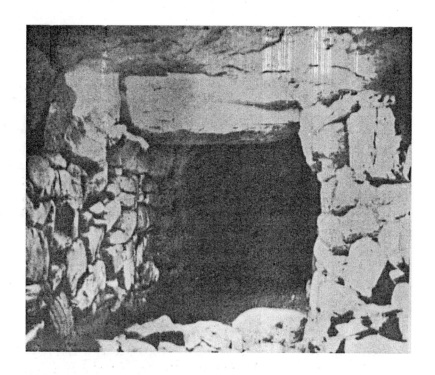

39. Inside the earth house at Kilkenneth, Tiree, 1916. (Nideck)

In Scotland, such barriers are uncommon, though the intention of such subterranea must have been as refuges. In South Uist the Uamh Sgalabhad has a large slab of rock brought from a different locality which serves to narrow the passage so as to render it almost impassable.

An account of an earth house discovered by accident in 1916 on the Isle of Tiree will serve to illustrate the typical features. In April 1916, John McIntyre, the tenant of a small farm at Kilkenneth in western Tiree, during ploughing hit a stone just beneath the surface which led to the discovery of an unsuspected earth house. Gilbert Goudie of the Society of Antiquaries of Scotland travelled to Tiree to investigate the find, and from his account we have McIntyre's description:

> In the month of April last (1916)1 was ploughing the ground for oats at the back of the house, about fifteen feet away, when the plough struck a small stone. I began to dig it out, and a lot more stones appeared immediately underneath. I thought this was the

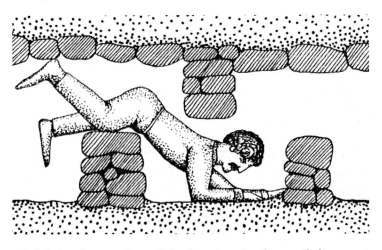

40. Mode of operation of the barriers in the earth house at Rathmullen, County Down, Ulster. (Nigel Pennick)

foundation of an old house, but when a few of the stones had been dug up I came upon what I found to be a lintel. On lifting it up, I found that there was below it an opening into the ground, so low that I could scarcely squeeze myself into it until some more earth had been removed. I got a candle and saw that this was the opening into a long passage. The opening was blocked up with lots of stones and earth. This I removed and cleared away for about three feet in past the entrance. I was then able to crawl onward for a long distance till I found the inner end was filled up the earth gradually sloping upwards until at the back it was about as high as the top of the side walls at the roof.

The earth house extended for about fifty feet. For a short distance from the entrance the direction of the tunnel is

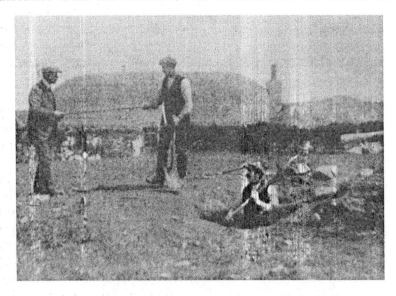

41. 1916 Photograph of the excavation of the earth house at Kilkenneth, Tiree. (Nideck)

southerly, then it bends with a curve to the south-east. Such abrupt bends are common features of earth houses and Fogous. The Tiree earth house has walls of well-fitted masonry laid in courses which converge towards the roof of the tunnel. Similar earth houses have been found elsewhere in Tiree and on other of the Western Isles: Lewis, Harris, Uist and Benbecula, and on the mainland in Aberdeen, Inverness, Perth, Forfar, etc. The largest known earth house is at Pitcur in Forfarshire near to Coupar Angus, which was described and illustrated by David MacRitchie in his privately published work *The Underground Life* (1892).

The age and use of earth houses has been long disputed. Some are certainly post-Roman, as they contain Roman masonry. The earth house at Crichton, Midlothian was found to have more than forty re-used Roman stones and when John Alexander Smith explored the earth house near the Roman fort at Newstead on Hadrian's Wall in 1845 he found worked stones, many of them bevelled on one edge. According to Joseph Anderson in *Scotland in Pagan Times* (1883), two of the stones have 'a rope-moulding of distinctly Roman character'.

Their use as dwellings is well-established. The tenth-century *Thorgil's Saga* refers to Thorgil and his men forcing their way into an earth house and encountering its inhabitants. Despite this early documentary evidence, respected writers like Thomas Pennant have dismissed the dwelling 'hypothesis'. In 1799 he wrote that earth houses were 'repositories for the ashes of sacrifice', as they had no ventilation and could scarcely be used for permanent dwellings. But more modern techniques of archaeology and the analysis of old manuscripts have revealed more than Pennant could have dreamt. An old manuscript referring to the Battle of Corcomroe in County Clare in 1317 speaks of Prince Donough summoning 'even every man in a caher's *souterrain*' to take part in the crucial battle.

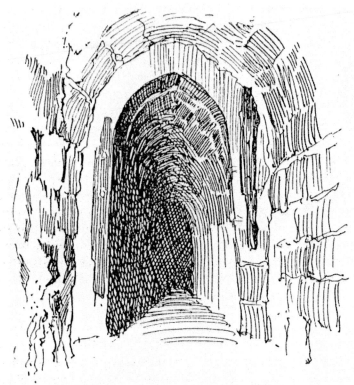

Secret Passage beneath Exeter.

42. Underground passages are the stuff of romance. (Nideck)

By 1868, John Stuart, addressing the Society of Antiquaries of Scotland, could assert: 'It has been doubted if these houses were ever really used as places of abode, a purpose for which they seem in no degree to be suited. But as to this there can be no real doubt. The substances found in many of them have been the accumulated debris of food used by man . . . in some cases the articles found would indicate that the occupation of these houses had come down to comparatively recent times.'

A parallel with life in these ancient subterranea is afforded by the Inuit earth houses which were in daily use until quite recently. In his book *Life With the Esquimaux,* published in 1864, Captain Hall wrote 'Formerly they built up an earth embankment, or a wall of stone about five feet high, and over this laid a skeleton of bones of the whale or spars of drift-wood, then on top of that placed skins of the seal or walrus... The entrances were serpentine tunnels under ground, with side walls, and roofed with slabs of stone. To pass through them one is obliged to go on "all-fours".' In the Aleutian Islands, the Inuit used to construct large earth house complexes which afforded shelter for up to one hundred families, but contact with modern civilization led to their abandoning this peculiar way of life.

The study of subterranea is often rendered difficult by changes in use. For example, there is evidence that the passage graves which are structurally related to earth houses and Fogous, may have only become tombs at a later date. Their astronomical orientation certainly indicates this. Evidence that earth houses were later used for burials comes from several sources. Sven Nilsson studied the gallery-huts and gallery-tombs of Scandivania and came to the conclusion that the tombs were copies of the houses. In *The Primitive Inhabitants of Scandinavia,* published in 1868 he wrote, 'We may rest assured that before the savage of the forest plains of Scania and West Gothland began to build gallery-chambers for the dead, he had already constructed similar ones for the living.' Sir Bertram Windle in *Life in Early Britain* (1897) observes that Sir Arthur Evans points out that early barrows of the north are in fact a copy of a primitive kind of mound-dwelling, such as is represented by the *gamme* of the Lapp.'

Among the Inuit of the Aleutian Islands there was a custom which resulted in their earth houses serving as both dwellings and tombs at the same time, for when a member of the community died, the body was walled up in the compartment which it had inhabited, and the rest of the tribe continued to live as before. The last known inhabitant of a Scottish earth house lived in one on the island of North Rona at the beginning of the last century. When they finally gave up living underground, the *uamh* finally passed into the province of history.

Deneholes

In various localities in Kent, Essex and Durham are found underground structures known as Deneholes. These often come to light as the result of a sudden subsidence, after which the usual course taken is to fill them in without further thought or investigation. Deneholes are very widespread, occurring almost everywhere that the underlying geology was favourable for their construction. They have been found in Essex at Grays, Chadwell and Tilbury, and in Kent at Aylesford, Bexley, Bexleyheath, Blackheath, Charlton, Cobham, Crayford, Darenth, Dartford, Dover, Erith, Faversham, Gillingham, Gravesend, Hammill, Hoo, Knockholt, Manston, Margate, Preston, Rochester, Rodmersham, Swanscombe, Woolwich, Wormshill and Yocklett's Bank. In Durham their localities and form are uncertain. Many of the Kentish and Essex deneholes have been explored during the last century, and a good idea of their structure and function has been gleaned from them.

The most thorough investigation of a group of deneholes was made between 1884 and 1887 by T. V. Holmes and W. Cole at

Hangman's Wood, Grays, Essex, where there are many deneholes in close proximity to one another. These pits vary in depth between seventy-eight and eighty-one feet, as compared with those in Kent which range from seventy feet at Dartford to 140 feet at Eltham. A typical denehole has a circular shaft about two feet six inches across, a suitable size for a person to descend by straddling opposite pairs of footholds which are still apparent in many deneholes. The shaft was sunk to a bed of chalk through an overburden of Thanet Sand. When chalk was reached, openings were excavated, and often a pattern known as the double trefoil was adopted. Sometimes, excavation of adjacent pits were joined, as at Hangman's Wood, for a pillared cavern facilitated the extraction of further chalk.

The Hangman's Wood explorers studied a group of eleven deneholes, some of which already opened into one another. Between them and other isolated deneholes the explorers drove connecting tunnels. Scale drawings were made and records taken of all the pits explored, and at certain places the Thanet Sand debris which is always found covering denehole floors was sifted for any remains which might indicate the age or origin of the pits.

Another group of deneholes investigated at about the same period was at Bexley in Kent, where F. C. J. Spurrell carried out intensive studies. In 1881 he published his findings in the *Archaeological Journal* in which he summarized all knowledge to date on the subject. For several years he had been studying deneholes all over the county, but concentrated on the large number which then existed in the largely rural area of Bexley. Today, Bexley is a suburban area of Greater London, and most of the woodland with deneholes has been built over.

Even in Spurrell's time, many deneholes had been filled in: 'On Crayford and Dartford Heath no caves remain now ... the

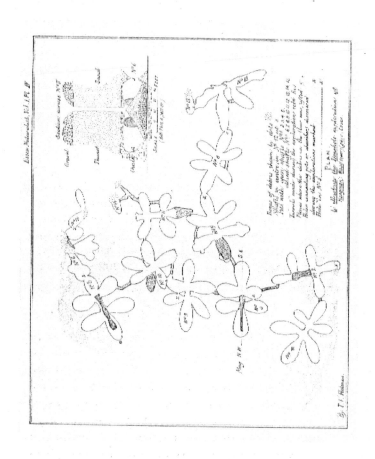

43. The denehole complex at Hangman's Wood, near Grays, Essex, England. Plan by T. V. Holmes, 1887. (Nideck)

places where they are most abundant is called Joyden's Wood and the copses around it.' In the area of Bexley there were three major clusters of deneholes: Stankey Wood, Cavey Springs and what is now known as Joyden's Wood. Spurrell claimed to have visited between thirty and forty deneholes in this area, most of which have been destroyed since his day. The 1910 Ordnance Survey Map of Stankey Wood marks twenty-five deneholes in an area of about five acres, and the overall number of pits in the Bexley district in the 1920s, before wholesale filling-in took place, was estimated to be in excess of 120.

The thirty-four deneholes at Cavey Springs were filled in during the late 1960s when the Central Electricity Generating Board constructed a power station there. Before building commenced, each denehole was located and filled with a slurry of Thanet Sand. Most of the deneholes in Joyden's Wood were likewise destroyed. Since the mid-1930s, housing developments in Bexley have encroached upon areas once woodland, and the only surviving deneholes in Joyden's Wood are in the southern sector where one very deep pit was not filled but instead was incorporated into the drainage system of a new housing estate.

Although Spurrell explored most of the Bexley deneholes in the 1880s, many more have subsequently come to light. In 1950, wet weather and subsequent subsidence led to the discovery of a typical denehole in the back garden of a house in Baldwyn's Park, where a vertical shaft opened to a depth of forty-five feet. At the bottom of this shaft was a set of chambers arranged in a double trefoil pattern, their walls and vaults bearing the roughly-hewn marks of miners' picks. The explorers of this pit, P. J. Tester and J. E. L. Caiger, noted that the tool marks visible on its walls were of rectangular section, similar to those made by modern tools. The use of metal picks of course rules out the romantic notion that all deneholes are of vast antiquity, for the tools used in the

151

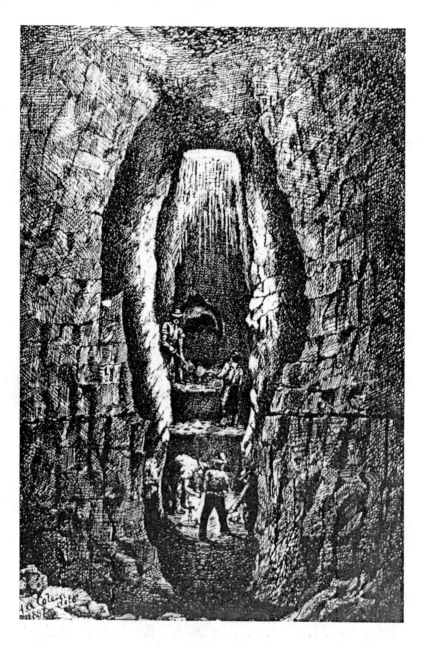

44. Inside a denehole. Drawing by H. G. Cole, 1887. (Nideck)

neolithic flint mines at Grimes Graves were no more than the antlers of deer, which make a shallower and more rounded impression.

The date of deneholes has long foxed archaeologists. As early as the first century of our era Pliny had written in his *Natural History* that chalk was extracted 'by means of pits sunk like wells, with narrow mouths, to the depth sometimes of one hundred feet, where they branch out like the veins of mines; and this kind is used chiefly in Britain'. They were certainly disused by 1570, however, when William Lambarde wrote of them in his *Perambulation of Kent*: 'There are to be seene, as well as in the open Heath neere to this Towne, as

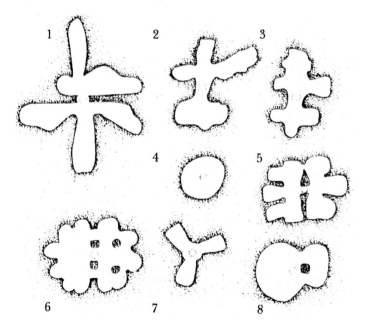

45. Kentish denehole plans: 1. Baldwyn's Park, Bexley; 2. Hammill; 3. Wingham Well; 4, 5, 6, Stankey Wood, Bexley; 7. Joyden's Wood, Bexleyt; 8. Stankey Wood, Bexley. (Nigel Pennick)

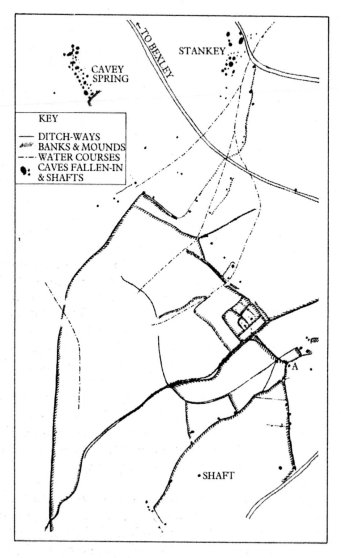

46. Spurrell's 1880 map of denehole distribution in Jordan's Wood, Bexley, Kent. (Nideck)

also in the closed Grounds about it, sundry artificial Caves, or Holes, in the Earth, whereof some have ten, some fifteene, some twenty fathoms in depth; at the Mouth (and thence downward) narrow, like to the Tonnell of a Chimney, or Passage of a Well; but in the bottom large, and of great receipt: insomuch as some of them have sundry Roomes (or Partitions) one within another, strongly vaulted and supported with Pillars of Chalke.'

Another early reference to them is found in Philemon Holland's translation of Camden's *Britannia*, published in 1610: 'Tilbury: neere unto which there be certaine holes in the rising of a Chalky Hill, sunke into the Grounde ten fathom deepe, the Mouth whereof is but Narrow, made of Stone cunningly wrought, but within they are Large and Spatious.' This edition is also of interest because it has the earliest illustration of deneholes, showing their long shafts and trefoil chambers. The Tilbury deneholes were at some time confused with the semi-legendary gold mines of Cymbeline. In his *Natural History of Oxfordshire*, published in 1705, Dr Robert Plot, commenting on the probable existence of metalliferous mines in that county, believed they must have been lost like 'the gold mines of Cunobeline in Essex, discovered again *temp.* Henry IV... and since lost again'. According to a correspondent in *The Cambrian Register* the gold mines at Orsett, East Tilbury, were being worked at the end of the fifteenth century. Later researchers, like Cole and Holmes who studied Hangman's Wood, thought that these references were garbled tales about the deneholes, though how they could have been mistaken for working gold mines is a mystery.

What, then, was the function of deneholes. They were certainly not sepulchral, though human remains, probably those of unsuspecting victims who fell in and died, have been discovered from time to time. Explorers like Spurrell, Cole and Holmes strove hard to solve this knotty problem by excavating the mounds of debris found at the bottom of the pits. Fragments of animal and human bones, smashed pottery of the fourteenth century and parts of millstones have been found at various times in debris cones, but such relics give few clues to the purpose of deneholes.

One of the most tenacious theories of the purpose of deneholes has been that of refuge in times of strife. Old writers, explaining the name 'denehole', invariably call it 'Dane-hole' allegedly from the period of the wars which culminated in the establishment of the Danelaw in Anglo-Saxon England. This etymological theory comes from a misinterpretation of the origin of the word, which derives from the Anglo-Saxon *denn*, a cave or pit. The supposed connection wiih the Danes was long believed proven. One of the strongest upholders of the refuge theory was the eminent antiquary W. H. D. Longstaffe who studied the deneholes in County Durham. In 1852, at a Newcastle meeting of the Archaeological Institute, Longstaffe read a paper entitled Durham before the Conquest. He claimed that the pits were formerly refuges used by Saxons

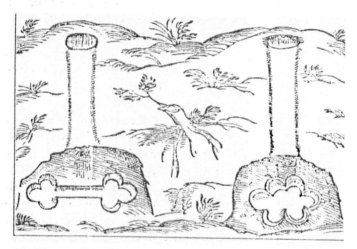

47. The earliest known representation of a denehole, from Camden's Britannia, 1610 edition. The deneholes at Tilbury, Essex. (Nideck)

fleeing from Danish marauders. 'They are frequent in Hartness,' he wrote, 'where the struggle seems to have been most bitter, and are described as excavations in the sides of eminences, in those sides from which the most extended views might be obtained.' These deneholes are unlike those in southern England in all but name, for they are excavated horizontally in magnesian limestone. They were formerly numerous on the coast and around Embleton, six miles west of Hartlepool.

Further evidence for the refuge theory was found at the bottom of a deep shaft in Eltham Park, Kent. The deepest denehole on record, 140 feet from top to bottom, it was examined by F. C.J. Spurrell and W. F. Petrie, the noted metrologist and Egyptologist. The shaft was steined with early sixteenth-century brickwork, and at the bottom was a chamber to one side of the shaft. This was supported by three pillars, and the single opening had been at some time concealed by a curtain indicated by iron pins which the archaeologists found still in place. These unique features led Spurrell to claim that the cavern had been a place of refuge during the sixteenth and seventeenth centuries, but although he acknowledged that some deneholes had served as shelters, he thought that that use was secondary, the deneholes having been built originally for the storage of grain.

Evidence that grain was stored underground in ancient Britain comes from the Greek historian and geographer Diodorus Siculus, who, on the evidence of the second century B.C. navigator Poseidonius, reported that the people of Britain had mean habitations and ate corn stored in underground pits. Spurrell's contention that these pits were deneholes came from a comparison with similar structures used in Spain and Morocco. Caesar and Tacitus noted the use of underground silos in northern France and Belgium, and the explorers of Hangman's Wood also held the theory that those deneholes were once granaries, mentioning the fragments of

157

millstone found there as corroborative evidence. Indisputable underground grain pits were once used in the Isle of Portland in Hampshire, but were of a different form than the denehole. They were beehive shaped pits walled with rubble-stone, and only about eight feet wide by twelve feet deep; in the bottom of one a considerable amount of black-ened corn was found, demonstrating their function. Holmes noted a strong

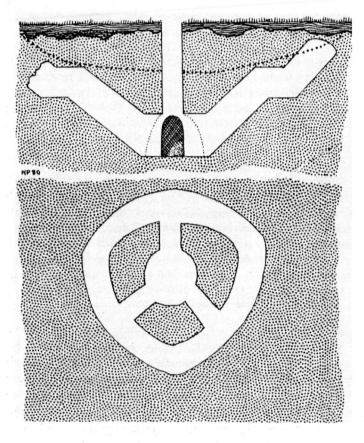

48. Section and plan of a Berkshire chalk well with a 20-foot shaft. Dotted line is 'dell' produced after collapse.
(Nigel Pennick)

resemblance between them and the rock-cut granaries of India.

The generally accepted theory now current for the function of deneholes is that they were primarily agricultural chalk mines for although chalk is the underlying stratum of many fields in the vicinity of deneholes, it has been known for centuries that a dressing of chalk improves the fertility of these fields. In times when transport was poor, it was only economic to dress fields with locally mined chalk, and deneholes proved the most acceptable method of providing it. They were dug in small, well-defined areas at the boundaries of fields, large numbers usually being made in close proximity to one another. Their design, which no doubt was handed down by experts to their apprentices, was evolved with the intention of maximizing output whilst producing a remarkably stable structure. When the denehole was finally abandoned as no longer productive, it was usually plugged with parts of trees and other agricultural debris, and then earth was shovelled on top of this makeshift plug. Naturally, the decay of timbers eventually leads to collapse, which nowadays means the rediscovery of a lost denehole.

From the fragments of pottery often found in deneholes and the proximity of the pits to medieval field boundaries, it is generally believed that most deneholes must date from the twelfth to the fifteenth centuries. After that date, techniques of mining agricultural chalk altered, and the chalk well was evolved. The mode of construction of these shafts was much nearer to the conventional water wells found everywhere, for the shaft was generally wider than in deneholes and was often steined with brickwork. The elegant and advanced techniques of denehole construction had degenerated into a much cruder and dangerous system. Unlike the carefully arranged self-supporting vaults of deneholes, chalk wells had rock domed chambers hacked out of the chalk, and often the span of these chambers was too wide for safety. The explorers of a chalk well at Nonington, Kent, discovered after subsidence of a lorry garage in 1939, found that the roof of the largest of four crude chambers had suffered a roof fall - a rare event in a denehole.

The Nonington chalk well was dated from the brick steining as eighteenth century. A more complex but nonetheless dangerous type of chalk well was studied by the geomantic researcher Francis J. Bennett who was in Berkshire and Buckinghamshire in 1887 where a highly-specialized form of chalk well was still in general use. 'Trial holes are dug, and the wells sunk, as far as possible, at the spots where the chalk is only just covered', wrote Bennett, 'When the required depth has been reached, what is termed 'angling' commences, i.e, headings are driven. These are level at first, but after a few yards they incline up towards the surface, which they almost reach, thus forming an inclined plane for the chalk hewn to run down into the boxes under the shaft ... After all the chalk wanted has been extracted, parts of the 'quoins' or divisions between the headings are usually knocked away . . . This causes the well to fall in, forming a "dell" or hollow at the surface of the ground.' The sign of an expert chalk-miner was to make the dell so shallow that it would not interfere with ploughing the field above.

In Bennett's time, such wells were in use to the north, north-east and west of Newbury and also in the southern parts of Buckinghamshire. Similar wells for lime were also once common, being made as deep shafts from which branched three galleries. Bennett measured two such wells, one at Basildon and the other at Hampstead Norris, both being sixty feet deep. The usual method for sealing a spent lime pit was more socially acceptable than the crude denehole plug, as bricklayers would be employed to seal them with strong brick caps as precautions against accident. All chalk mining and lime pit working was discontinued round about the beginning of World War I and such arts can now be considered dead.

Even today there are new discoveries waiting to be made. The function of deneholes has still not been conclusively proved, and the information gleaned over a century of explanation is scattered in the obscure pages of learned journals and rare monographs. As further deneholes subside beneath roads and gardens, garage forecourts and private houses, new exploration may shed some new light upon this puzzling enigma.

Chapter Nine

Eccentrics

English Eccentrics Underground

The possession of almost unlimited resources often lead their owners into undertaking extraordinary extravagances. In former times, the landed gentry and capitalist barons of England created what to-day can be recognized as works of art in the form of non-utilitarian buildings and constructions that went by the collective name of 'follies'. The seventeenth and eighteenth century love of classical ruins led to the construction of new ones, geomantically placed in the landscape according to the principles of picturesque painting and the conventions of Chinese feng-shui in its anglicized form as Sharawadgi. The eighteenth-century pagoda in Kew Gardens, London, is the most notable example of this early integration of feng-shui and English landscape gardening. All over the country, 'Roman', 'Gothick', 'Chinoise' and 'Rustick' follies graced the enclosed private estates of the rich. These were the visible instances of 'follies'. There were (and are) others, burrowed invisibly in the ground.

Perhaps the earliest undergound 'follies' were made in the seventeenth century. Military tunnelling in the English Civil War had been honed to a fine art, having assimilated perfectly Renaissance understanding of both engineering, surveying and a subtle understainding of landscape. The remains of tunnels made during the siege of Bridgnorth, Shropshire, by Cromwell's engineers can still be seen. It was in the south of England, in Surrey, with its existing tradition of stone-mining (as at Chaldon), that 'folly tunnelling' began. William Harvey (died 1657) had artificial caves excavated in his garden at Combe, Surrey, so that he could meditate in peace. Henry Howard, Duke of Norfolk, had a 'crypta' dug by George and John Evelyn at his estate at Albury Park in the mid-1600s. This was a tunnel over 150 yards in length, containing a subterranean 'Roman Bath' dated 1676.

In his *Brief Lives*, John Aubrey wrote of the tunnels that Charles Howard made at Deepdene, Dorking, Surrey: "In the hill....is a cave digged thirty six paces long, and five yards high; and at about two thirds of the hill (where the crook, or bowing, is) he hath dug another subterranean walk or passage, to be pierced through the hill; through which as through a tube you have the vista over all the south part of Surrey and Sussex to the sea. The south side of this hill is converted into a vineyard of many acres of ground which faceth the south and south west. The vaulting or upper part of those caves are not made semicircular, but parabolical, which is the strongest figure for bearing and which sandy ground naturally falls into then stands. And thus we may see that the conies (by instinct of Nature) make their holes so."

Beginning in 1718, the poet Alexander Pope tunnelled beneath both his own property and the road that separated his garden from his house in Twickenham. Pope's friends visited Wookey Hole in Somerset and shot down stalactites to adorn his tunnel. Mirrors, shells, amethysts, 'Cornish diamonds', 'Brazilian pebbles' and quartz crystals completed the decor. Pope sat in the tunnel, with his back to the door, and watched the word go by by means of precisely-located mirrors. When the doors were closed, the tunnel became a *camera obscura*, on the wall of which was projected the scene outside.

At Clifton in Bristol in the mid-1700s, Thomas Goldeney made tunnels. In his *Memorandum*, he notes that in 1737, he

163

"finished the Subterraneous Passage to the Grotto and began upon the Grotto in the same year". It took him until 1764 to finish the Grotto, complete with its decoration of sea shells. He made an artificial spring, powered by a 'fire-engine', (an atmospheric engine, forerunner of the steam engine). Its waters issued from an urn held by a marble image of the god Neptune.

Sometimes 'folly tunnelling' was done to conceal activities of which 'public opinion' disapproved. The Hell-Fire Caves at West Wycombe (see below) are such an example. There, Sir Francis Dashwood and his aristocratic co-orgiasts could cavort to their satanic and sexual hearts' content. The frisson of entering the underworld to partake of the pleasures and terrors of Hades could not be achieved in any other way. Other rich folly-builders constructed 'Committee Rooms', as at Ware in Hertfordshire, Chapels and Ballrooms, as at Welbeck Abbey in Nottinghamshire, or rooms with no discernable purpose, such as those beneath Liverpool.

One of the greatest of tunnelling eccentrics was 'The Mole of Mason Street', Joseph Williamson. Williamson was a 'self-made man', born poor in 1769, but, through astute business acumen, and a favourable marriage, he became rich. On his retirement in 1818, he began to tunnel beneath his house in Mason Street, Edge Hill, Liverpool. Williamson "appears to have been a true Troglodyte, one who preferred the Cimmerian darkness of his vaulted world, to the broad cheerful light of day". After his retirement, he lived in a cellar, and slept in a vaulted cave. From the cellar, a heavy wooden door gave access to a maze of tunnels that he extended continuously throughout the rest of his life. To-day, he would be called a performance artist. He died in 1841.

His tunnels were made by workmen whom he employed, as a form of relief in times when no other work was available. Williamson said that his prime motive was "the employment of the poor;. for if you give them something to do, no matter what, it keeps them out of mischief". Williamson made no profit from the tunnels. The stone that they dug out was not sold. St Jude's church in Liverpool was constructed of stone from one of Williamson's tunnels, donated free of charge. Williamson appears to have hated requests from the curious to view his tunnels, replying to them that they were not "show-shops, nor was he a showman". In 1834, when the railway engineers under the direction of Stephenson were building the Edge Hill tunnel, they broke into one of Williamson's tunnels and saw the man himself with his labourers. It is said that he told the astonished navvies that he was 'The King of Edge Hill' and that he could show them how to tunnel if they wanted to learn a lesson in that "polite art".

The only survey of the tunnels ever made was undertaken by Dr George C. Watson, who wrote under the pseudonym of 'Medicus'. He was given a pass by Williamson, which read: "Dr. Watson is not to be interrupted in his walks on my premises, either on the surface, or under the surface. January, 1839. J.W.". Watson stated that the tunnels were perfect marvels, not only for their great extent, but for the excellence of their construction, and their inapplicability to any possible purpose. After Joseph Williamson's death, attempts were made to explore the tunnels. In 1844, explorers discovered a cave, between 30 and 40 feet in width, about 60 feet beneath the surface. Massive and complex brick vaulting supported the roof. Because of the perceived danger, most of the tunnels were bricked up, or their entrances filled with rubble. "Eccentric or unaccountable-looking arches" as they were described not long afterwards are never looked upon favourably by the city fathers!

As the writer of *The Streets of Liverpool* noted: "His costly excavations and galleries are now filled up, his vaults are destroyed or covered over, and his great delf is a tradition.

Had he spent his money usefully on the surface, instead of uselessly under it, those who came after him would have doubtless had more satisfaction".

Chapter Ten

Notable Subterranea of Britain

Thousands of places in Britain have tunnels or legends of tunnels, and space precludes a comprehensive gazetteer - it would run to thousands of entries. Some places, however, have subterranea of special note, either for their extent, their unique features or their historical and legendary associations. This section explores the most notable and interesting examples in Britain.

Glastonbury

Reputed as the place of the earliest Christian foundation in Britain, Glastonbury has several reputed tunnels whose whereabouts were investigated by the psychic archaeologist Frederick Bligh Bond at the beginning of this century. There are five main tunnel stories attached to the Abbey, and three have been in some measure verified.

The first tunnel leads from the medieval George and Pilgrim Inn to a point within the Abbey grounds. Built by Abbot Selwood in about 1470, the tunnel may have been intended as a secret access to the Abbey for visitors to the Inn. The tunnel begins at the south end of the inn's cellar under the High Street and is clear for twenty feet until it encounters a more modern sewer; from there it is assumed that the passage continues to the Abbot's Gateway, where there was formerly a porter's lodge, but this has not been verified by excavation. A

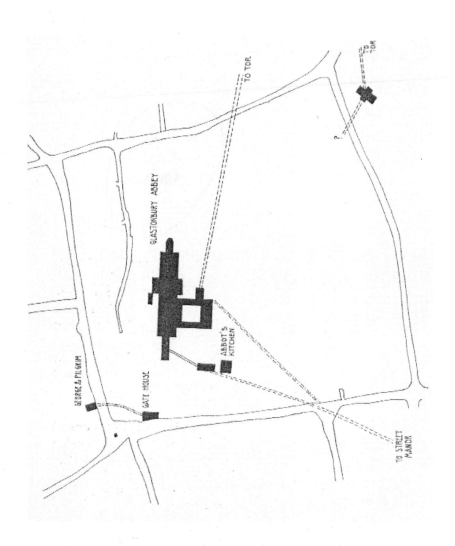

*49. Real, legendary and reputed tunnels around the Abbey
ruins at Glastonbury, Somerset, England. (Nigel Pennick)*

trip along this tunnel is described by Mrs Bilbrough in her diary of 21 May 1918, quoted in Alan Fea's *Rooms of Mystery and Romance*. 'Off we started on our underground journey down a flight of fearfully steep steps, dark and damp and slippery ... We groped our way to where the far-famed passage was, which had a great stone step at the entrance, and was only three feet in height, so that those who used it must have crawled on their nees, resting at intervals where ledges are cut in the sides for that purpose. Fancy going for a quarter mile like that, when even a few feet of it made my back ache and my limbs quiver all over from the unnatural strained position.'

Bond described the passage as 'a low tunnel formed in well-cut stone with a pointed segmental roof, and furnished on each side with a projecting stone ledge, for an elbow-rest'.

A second tunnel is alleged to lead from the crypt of the Lady Chapel beneath the River Brue to some distant point, probably in the village of Street where a passage is known to run from an outbuilding in the grounds of the old Manor House. It is said that a dog was once put into the tunnel at Street. It emerged later at Glastonbury Abbey. The passage at Street cannot be explored for any distance as it is blocked; at the Abbey end Bond excavated the reputed site of the tunnel but found the subsoil totally unsuitable for tunnelling.

Another passage was remembered to Bond by an old inmate of the Women's Almshouse who said that in her childhood a passage was known running from the well chamber at the south side of the Galilee. A lamb once fell into the hole and was lost, occasioning the sealing of the tunnel. Bond cut a trench around the chamber, which ran through the monks' graveyard to a point nearly due south of the well in the crypt. The rubble at this point gave way to a trench filled with clay, which suggests that a tunnel once ran there. It may have run southwards across the graveyard towards the Guest Hall and

Almonry, and may have been connected with services in the crypt. It provided a covered way from the monastic buildings to the crypt, enabling the monks to gain access to the shrine undetected by pilgrims and sheltered from the weather and prying eyes.

The third tale is of a large underground passage in the field to the south of the Abbey. There was once a subsidence there which revealed the stone head of a channel, and an old workman named Thyer told Bond that he remembered having seen a deep-walled passage with flagstones opened by the then owner of the Abbey, Mr Austin. When Bond attempted to locate the passage, Thyer was unable to remember the exact location. Yet another tunnel was said to have existed to the south of the Abbot's Kitchen, being a stone- built channel which crossed the orchard to a point on the Abbey's western boundary.

During excavations for the footings of the Abbot's House, a trench was dug running to the south-east of the Refectory. The main drain of the Abbey was revealed here a little beyond the southernmost boundary of the Abbot's House. One of Bond's students entered this passage and climbed along it for some sixty feet before encountering an obstruction. The drain ran in a south-westerly direction to the lowest point of Magdalene Street where once stood a chain bridge and probably a water-gate to the Abbey for access of barges.

A fourth tunnel is a reputed to go from the Abbey to the Tor, or more specifically to the now-ruined St Michael's church which surmounts that most majestic of Somerset landmarks. The Tor itself is reputed to be undermined with a warren of tunnels, with a large entrance located somewhere near the waterworks reservoir in Wellhouse Lane. Many dowsers have felt that the Tor is honeycombed with passages, but none of these have yet been located.

The fifth tunnel is said to begin eight miles from Glastonbury Tor at a collection of ancient megaliths called the Deerleap Stones. As usual, the legendary dog was put into the tunnel only to be found some days later wandering on Glastonbury Tor. Two tunnels which have no associated legends were discovered by accident in 1974 when a heavy vehicle crashed through the road surface at the main entrance to the Abbey Barn during some filming there. A large tunnel was revealed which ran in the direction of the Abbey Refectory, but before it could explored, it was filled in with rubble by the contracters who at that time were engaged in repairing the ancient barn. Another subterranean passage was revealed at the same time, running towards the Tor, but this, too, suffered the same fate.

West Wycombe, Buckinghamshire

The exploits of the eighteenth-century Hell Fire Club are still notorious today. The satanic club was founded by the wealthy rake Sir Francis Dashwood and counted among its members a Prime Minister, the Chancellor of the Exchequer, the Lord Mayor of London, many great artists, writers and poets, and even a son of the Archibishop of Canterbury. They were all dedicated to the practice of Satanism and sexual license, and as a setting for conspiracies and orgies of the cult, Dashwood in 1752 purchased the remains of the Abbey of Medmenham, founded in 1160. The organization he founded was overtly magical, being called the Friars of St Francis of Wycombe, and Dashwood reconstructed the abbey and its surroundings to enhance their activities.

The chapel of the abbey was furnished with a pornographic ceiling, and stained glass depicting the sexual acts of the Friars. In the gardens were many statues with a sexual theme, and among the shrubbery Dashwood made an artificial grotto which he dubbed the Cave of Trophonius, after the Classical cave 'from whence all creatures came out melancholy', a Dashwood conceit explained in a Latin inscription over its entrance: 'All animals after sexual inter-

171

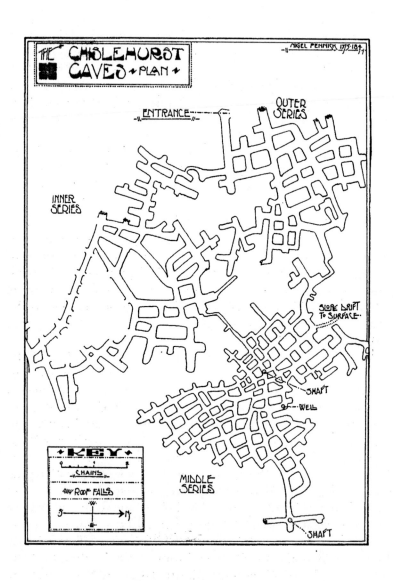

50. The Chislehurst Caves, as in 1975. (Nigel Pennick)

course feel melancholy except the barnyard cock or those who love to give it away.'

The grotto, now called the Hell Fire Caves, was built by foreign workmen imported specially for the purpose then packed off home when the work was complete. Cut into a chalk cliff, the caves sport grotesque carvings of devil's heads, and a cursing well in which the High Priestesses were baptized. An underground stream encountered during construction was dubbed the River Styx, and, like its counterpart in the Oracle of the Dead at Baiae, was used in initiatory rites. The caves are now open to the public, and prove an irresistible attraction.

Kent

The county of Kent is of especial interest to students of subterranea, for its geology is ideal for the digging of deneholes, caves and tunnels. Of all the many Kentish subterranea, the caves at Chislehurst are the most extensive, though the early history of Chislehurst gives no clues to the origin of this remarkable network.

The revival of antiquarian interest during the middle of the last century led to the study of local curiosities all over Britain, and the Chislehurst Caves naturally attracted considerable attention. By the middle of the nineteenth century their use, let alone their origin, was shrouded in mystery. One of the first explorers of the network was W. J. Nichols. 'After proceeding with difficulty', he wrote, he was obliged to abandon the attempt: even where exploration was not absolutely impracticable, clambering over huge masses of chalk in semi-darkness was decidedly dangerous, and there was the further risk of losing the right track amid the tortuous windings of the place.' On enquiring locally, Nichols determined from the 'oldest inhabitant of the locality' that the caves had been closed in about 1800, but no further information was forthcoming.

But just what are the caves? Many theories have been advanced to account for these tunnels, which ramify under an area of about twenty acres. Visitors to the caves today will be regaled with stories of Druidic rites and sacrifice, but the origins appear more prosaic. When Nichols first explored the caves in about 1860 he noticed that the walls of the system, which is divided into three main 'series', were expertly tooled. To those accustomed to modern mining techniques, such tooling was baffling. This led to the theory that the tunnels were not abandoned mine workings, but the hypogeal shrines of the ancient Druids. 'That they are not merely galleries formed for the purpose of obtaining chalk and flints', wrote Nichols, 'must be apparent to any visitor who will devote a few minutes to their examination: they are regularly formed, symmetrical, and in many places very beautiful in their curved and well-proportioned outlines. The finishing-work, too, has been executed with a due regard to evenness, particularly in the dressing of the lower walling, which has been done with a finely-pointed wrought-iron pick with a slightly curved angular blade.'

From these observations, Nichols concluded that the caves were certainly religious in function, as he believed the ancient Celtic priesthood had used such extensive hypogea in their rites. 'These hypogeal works are so extensive that temple, seminary, storehouse and refuge, each to a certain extent distinct from the other, may at one and the same time have been included in them.'

Such enthusiasm was not shared by two mining experts who studied the cave system during 1904. R. E. and R. H. Forster examined the finishing work of the tunnels and concluded that it was characteristic of the work of the Northumberland pitmen of the early eighteenth century. 'The middle series of workings in particular bear so strong a resemblance to some of the Old High Main coal workings in the neighbourhood of Newcastle that it is possible to conjecture that this portion

174

has been worked under the management of an expert pitman from that district', concluded the Forsters. Their conclusion is reinforced by the observation that the lime-kilns of Kent, from the seventeenth century onwards, were fired by coal brought down the coast from Newcastle.

Another prominent feature of the caves was seen by Nichols as evidence of unspeakable rites. At the end of almost every unfinished working in the Chislehurst Caves are the so-called 'Druids' Altars', about which he waxed lyrical: 'We see one of the most interesting sights that these caves can show us; a series of galleries with rectangular crossings, containing many chambers of semi-circular, or apsidal form, to the number of thirty or more - some having "altar-tables" formed in the chalk, within a point or two of true orientation.' These 'altars' are in reality the remains of 'bottom canch working', a well-known tunnelling technique in which the upper part of the tunnel is removed first, leaving a lower step or shelf, the 'bottom canch', on which the miner stands as he drives the tunnel forwards. When the tunnel is sufficiently deep, the bottom canch is taken up. By these methods the Chislehurst miners excavated tunnels up to twelve feet high and fifteen feet wide, narrowing. The method of mining used here is known elsewhere variously as 'stoop and room' or 'post and stall'. Used in early coal mines, it was soon abandoned for more economical methods of working such as 'board and wall' which extracted more coal with equal safety, but it was ideal for the more extensive strata of chalk.

The Chislehurst Caves are in reality three separate mines linked together by irregular tunnels which seem to have been driven from the middle workings in order to test the positions of the other two workings. This demonstrates some skill in underground surveying, but does not rule out an early date; however, the boundaries of the workings, which terminate at the road up Chislehurst Hill, show that the mining was carried out within well-defined limits which seems a recent concept. Like most abandoned subterranea, the caves have seen re-use.

When Nichols explored them in about 1860, he found piles of flint, the remains of flint-knapping for the muskets which would have been used to defend Britain if Napoleon I had invaded. In 1871 the caves had another Napoleonic connection when the deposed Emperor Napoleon III used part of them as a store for his rescued possessions.

Even if Nichols was mistaken about the former uses of the caves as 'temple, seminary, storehouse, and refuge', the events of the 1940s proved him strangely prophetic. 'It was in the Second World War when the caves really came to the fore', wrote Ann Pennick in *Deneholes and Subterranea.* 'They were the first and most important air raid shelter in Great Britain. The owner opened his caves to the public, mostly women and children, but also some men who were taking a well-earned rest from the Blitz in London.' Up to 15,000 people made their nightly home in the cave system, and a virtual subterranean town was created for them.

Various parts of the caves were adapted as shops, a gymnasium, dance hall, cinema, canteens and even a church. At the height of their use, it is reported that the canteens provided over 300 gallons of tea nightly to the thirsty shelterers. Sanitary, medical and washing facilities were naturally installed in the subterranean shelters, and a baby was even born there. She was christened Cavina in the underground church.

Chislehurst is not the only cave system in Kent. At Eastry there was an extensive system referred to in W. F. Shaw's *History of Eastry,* published in 1870. In it he wrote: 'The cave was of comparatively modern origin, having been excavated by a previous owner of the property, a Mr Foord, a builder. Mr Solley is inclined to think that it was accidentally discovered by Foord when excavating chalk, and that he made the steps down to it ... He may have preferred to have claimed it as his own handiwork rather than his discovery.'

The cave consisted of a maze of narrow passages at varying depths beneath the surface, and it was possible to walk round and come back to the well at a lower level. One part of the complex was enlarged into a small chamber which was given the name of the church'. At the far end of this chamber was a crude figure carved out of the chalk. Similar figures exist at Royston and existed in one entrance to the Chislehurst Caves until defaced by shelterers during World War II.

Another system of abandoned mines exists beneath Hosey Common at Westerham in Kent. The age of these mines is unknown, but they were constructed for the extraction of a special sandstone known as Kentish Ragstone. Four seperate complexes have been explored, but they are sealed with strong gates as they support a large bat population.

Although it is now much run down, the naval dockyard at Chatham was once a vital link in the nation's defences. In an area most likely to suffer invasion, a system of fortifications consisted of various batteries of artillery, defensive strongpoints, barracks and other military necessities. One of the forts in this chain defences is Fort Amherst, below which lies a system of tunnels which are an expansion of more ancient workings, a chalk well and a man-made cave of uncertain date and function. The cave began in a quarry now known as the Cave Yard, and during the last years of the eighteenth and the first years of the nineteenth it was enlarged and extended to connect with a series of underground gun emplacements which overlook a vast defensive ditch.

The tunnels are still penetrable for over half a mile. Remains of military equipment from the Napoleonic to the nuclear age

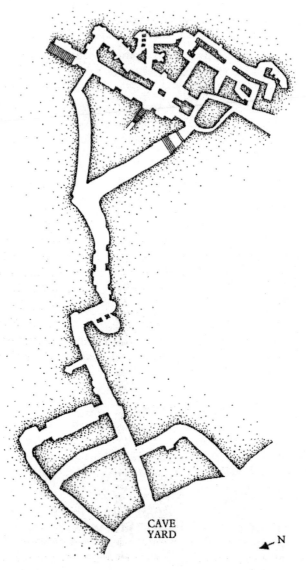

CAVE
YARD

N

*51. Tunnels leading from Cave Yard under Fort Amherst,
Chatham, Kent. (Nigel Pennick)*

lie about abandoned, relics including bed frames from World War II when the cave served as an air-raid shelter. Various flights of steps and hoist shafts link the tunnels with the upper part of the battery and defences. During the summer of each year between the end of the Napoleonic Wars and the outbreak of World War I, military exercises added to the network of tunnels so that now a massive uncharted jumble of tunnels extends beneath the hills around Chatham, and, being makeshift , are extremely dangerous. One of these exercises is recorded by local author Charles Dickens in *The Pickwick Papers.*

During the eighteenth century it was considered the height of fashion to construct shell grottoes in the grouns of stately homes, a harmless variation on the sinister machinations of the Dashwood set. These shell grottoes had their origin in a old English custom which has now quite died out. Each summer, on or about 25 July, children would fashion small 'grottoes' from mud, sticks or wood, and adorn them with oyster-shells to beg for money off passers-by as they still do around Guy Fawkes Day, the old Pagan festival of *Samhain*. A traditional rhyme accompanied the making of these grottoes, which were sacred to St James (Sant'Iago) of Compostella:

> Please remember the Grotto,
> It's only once a year,
> Father's gone to sea,
> And Mother's gone to fetch him back,
> So please remember me!
> A penny won't hurt you-
> Tuppence won't put you in the workhouse!

All over the country, the remains of shell grottoes moulder neglected in the grounds of once-great country mansions, but at Margate the most spectacular and famous of them all is still in good repair and accessible to the public. A strange

179

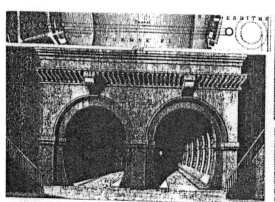
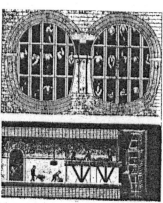
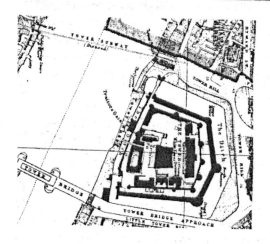
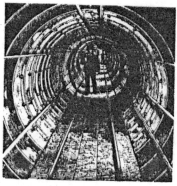

cross- and circular- shape, its odd form has inevitably led speculation about its origin, but the eighteenth century shell cladding prevents further investigation.

London

As a city, London has existed for the best part of two millennia so it is not surprising that there are many subterranean structures concealed beneath the city streets. Owing to the continuous reconstruction of the city over the centuries, however, the number of ancient and mysterious structures are few in comparison with the sewers, cable tunnels, underground railways and air raid shelters of modern times.

Many of the ancient rivers and streams which used to cross the city of London or the farmland outside the city walls have been relegated into sewers canalized ignominiously below ground in pipes. Among these are the Tyburn, which gives its name to the infamous place of execution, now Marble Arch; the Cranbourne, still marked by a street name near Leicester Square; the Ravensbourne, the Walbrook, the Effra Brook, the Westbourne and the Fleet. Place names like Knightsbridge and Holborn are now the only indications that there were once streams at those places. Many of these former streams are now integrated with the vast sewer system developed over the last three hundred years and perfected during the last century.

There are many ancient crypts beneath the churches of London, and some which have outlived the churches for which

---

Opposite: 52. Earl subriver tunnels in London. Above: Route, portals and constructional techniques of the first subaqueous tunnel, between Rotherhithe and Wapping. Below: Route and view inside the Tower Subway, the world's first tube railway (1869) (Nideck)

they were built. When the old church of St Mary Le Bow was burnt with much of London in 1666, Sir Christopher Wren was commissioned to build anew on the site. During demolition of the ruins, Wren discovered beneath the old church a barrel-vaulted crypt which had been forgotten for centuries. Probably the oldest surviving structure in London, it was stated by Stow in his *Survey of London* that the church was formerly called *de arcubus* or 'of the arches' because 'in the reign of William the Conqueror' it was 'the first in the city built on arches of stone'.

Although now subterranean, this arched structure once stood at street level. From at least 1172, the ecclesiastical Court of Arches was held at St Mary Le Bow, and several commentators have suggested that it may be far older than the twelfth century, perhaps being of the same date as the crypt, which some believe Roman. When Wren rebuilt the church, he carried out his own excavations of the crypt and found a door which opened, eighteen feet beneath street level, onto a Roman roadway whose paving was still intact.

The Tower of London of course has several tunnel legends, as do both St Paul's Cathedral and Westminster Abbey. Tunnels are reputed to run beneath Hampstead Heath and Clapham Common, and a modern legend tells of a tunnel running from Buckingham Palace to Heathrow Airport, presumably for the monarch's escape in time of war. It is the most modern addition to the traditional tales of tunnels attached to notable buildings.

The terrain under London is mainly gravels and clays, ideal for tube railways but unproductive in mining terms, so there are few ancient mines under London on a Parisian scale. However, during 1946 a collapse under Alliance Road in Woolwich revealed some ancient chalk mines built between 1850 and 1914 to extract material used as a flux in brick making. The workings originally were eight feet wide at floor

182

level and fifteen feet in height, but the fall in the water table owing to the extraction of water from boreholes from the end of the nineteenth century enabled the miners to re-work the tunnels and mine another five feet of chalk from the floors. After a survey of the general state of the old mines, they were filled in as a potential hazard.

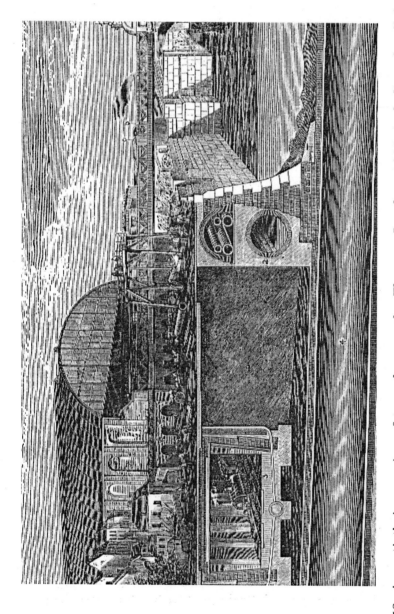

53. An artist's impression of tunnels near the Thames, London, 1867, including the ill-fated Whitehall and Waterloo pneumatic railway. (Nideck)

Chapter Eleven

Tunnels Under London

To-day, the extensive deep underground rail system of London is the backbone of passenger transport in the Metropolis. The small profile trains that run through the tube tunnels are an indispensible part of the London scene, and have been for more than a century. All of this is possible only because of the geology that underlies the city streets. Beneath the greater part of the city, from Hampstead in the north to Kennington in the south, and from the City of London in the east to beyond Hammersmith in the west, is a thick stratum known as the London Clay. This is a homogeneous sedimentary deposit, laid down seventy million years ago as a fluid mud. Over the aeons, the enormous pressure exerted by overlying strata reduced the clay's water content, compacting the fine particles into a stiff, overconsolidated and impermeable mass. This clay bed fills the great geological depression known as the London Basin, where it is encountered between ten and thirty feet beneath the ground surface. At the margins of the London Basin, it is very thick: 400 feet at Wimbledon and 300 feet at Highgate; whilst at the centre it is much thinner, ranging from 70 to 100 feet. It has been lost completely from Hackney, parts of the City of London, the area around Tottenham Court Road, Rotherhithe, Deptford, Greenwich and Woolwich.

The London Clay is an excellent material through which to tunnel, though it varies a little in its composition. Tunnelling through the pure clay is relatively easy, for it is far softer than

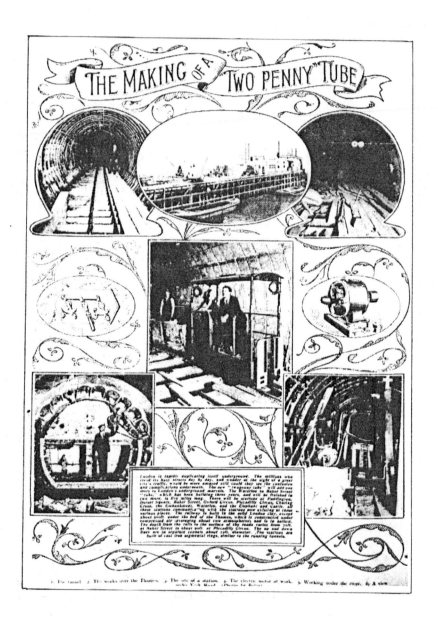

THE MAKING OF A "TWO PENNY" TUBE

London is rapidly duplicating itself underground. The millions who crowd its busy streets day by day, and wonder at the sight of a great city's traffic, would be more amazed still could they see the confusion and complications underneath. The new "twopenny tube" will add one more to London's underground marvels. The Waterloo to Baker Street "tube," which has been building three years, and will be finished in two more, is five miles long. There will be stations at Paddington, Dorset Square, Baker Street, Oxford Circus, Piccadilly Circus, Charing Cross, the Embankment, Waterloo, and the Elephant and Castle, all these stations communicating with the stations now existing at these various places. The railway is built in the mild London clay, except about 300ft. under the bed of the Thames, which is constructed under compressed air averaging about two atmospheres, and is in ballast. The depth from the rails to the surface of the road varies from 30ft. at Baker Street to about 90ft. at Piccadilly Circus. The up and down lines are in separate tunnels about 12ft. diameter. The stations are built of cast iron segmental rings, similar to the running tunnels.

1. The tunnel. 2. The works over the Thames. 3. The site of a station. 4. The electric motor at work. 5. Working under the river. 6. A view under York Road. (Photos by Roburn)

solid rock and impervious, so no water is ever encountered in it. But its elasticity can cause problems, especially on the surface, for tunnelling sets up movements in the clay ahead of the tunnel face. This has been known to cause settling and other movements in buildings perhaps a hundred feet above. Also, on exposure to the air, London Clay loses its elasticity and tends to disintegrate. In some places, the clay may contain pockets of other material: beneath old watercourses, for instance, the clay may be what is known as short or rotten. In these places, tunnelling is considerably more difficult. Beneath the clay lie the Woolwich and Reading Beds, a mixture of coloured sands, clays, shelly deposits, concretions, flint and quartz pebbles. Known as Shepherd's Plaid, these beds range from 25 to 80 feet in thickness, are water-bearing, and outcrop between Dulwich, Plumstead and Eltham. Materials such as these have been encountered during the construction of tube railways under London, and appropriate measures, detailed later, have been necessitated to deal with them.

Because of the special qualities of the London Clay, special methods of tunnelling deep underground railways were developed during the nineteenth century. The first underground railway construction anywhere was the extension of the London and Birmingham Railway from Chalk Farm to Euston Square, which opened in 1838. This ran for $1^{1}/_{8}$ miles from Regent's Canal to Euston Square, comprising 1526 yards of covered way and cutting. The first true section of underground railway was the 310 yards of covered way on the L&BR, built by the cut-and-cover technique, roofed by

---

Opposite: 54. An advertisement issued during the construction of the Baker Street and Waterloo Railway, London (now the central section of the Bakerloo Line) circa 1902. (Electric Traction Publications

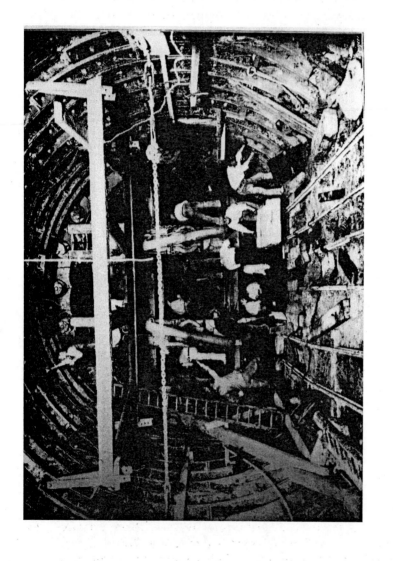

55. 'Tunnel Tigers' working at the tunnel face during the construction of a tube railway under London, circa 1900. (Electric Traction Publications)

crescent-shaped cast-iron girders. Because it was built for a mainline railway, this pioneer section is rarely credited as the true origin of subterranean metropolitan railways. The accolade of the first is always given to the first fully urban underground railway or Metro, the Metropolitan Railway, which was also built in London to link Paddington with King's Cross. It opened in 1863. The disruption to street traffic and trade caused by its construction by the cut-and-cover method - digging an enormous trench in the street, lining the walls with brick, then arching it over to create a running tunnel - had occasioned much criticism. Streets were closed in sections 200 yards long for up to four months at a time, and traffic diverted. Only a year after the Metropolitan opened, a Joint Committee of Parliament, considering the future of urban railways, pronounced against temporary openings and shafts in the road, so alternative methods had to be sought if new lines were to be built. Of course, London had an eminent precedent for deep-level tunnel construction - the first purpose-built under-river tunnel ever made. This was the celebrated Thames Tunnel engineered by the French genius Sir Marc Brunel.

This pioneering tunnel was built with great difficulty: strikes, roof falls and floods all played their part in prolonging the construction period, which lasted eighteen years and twenty-three days in all from 1825 until 1843. A major project which many believed impossible, the tunnelling aroused constant interest, and when something went wrong, knowing pronouncements from the "I told you so" brigade, who then, as now, awaited disaster with glee. In 1827, the Curate of Rotherhithe, from whose parish the tunnel was being constructed, announced in a sermon that a flooding of the tunnel was "a just judgement of the Almighty on the presumptuous aspirations of mortal men". *The Times* was a notable opponent of the tunnel, and also opposed the Waterloo and City Railway sixty years later. Despite the religious objections, the tunnel was finished, though its misfortunes, engineering and financial, were to affect the financial prospects of later subaqueous projects in the Metropolis.

Brunel's tunnel was pioneering in more ways than one. Apart from being the first purpose-built under-river crossing, it was the first tunnel driven with a tunnelling shield. In his Patent (No. 4204 of 1818), Brunel described an apparatus "intended to precede the body or shell of the tunnel", thus preventing any collapse of the material through which the tunnel was being driven. Brunel, who had been instigator of several major innovations in shipyard practice, had followed Nature and taken his idea from a pest familiar in the days of wooden vessels, the Shipworm, *Teredo navalis,* which bores its own living tunnels through hard wood in seawater.

The other advance in tunnelling technique necessary for the genesis of the tube railway was not employed by Brunel, who used traditional brick lining. Brick linings are neither rapidly erected, nor suitable for tunnels through certain classes of material. Eventually, Brunel used a shield to create tunnels of the traditional arch form which is far easier to make in brick than a cylindrical one. The ideal material for a tunnel driven by a cylindrical shield was cast iron, being relatively cheap, durable and in ready supply. Although civil engineers were late to use cast iron, the mine engineers, pioneers in every way, had used it as early as 1796. In that year, 'tubbing in circles' - cast iron rings - had been used to line the shaft of Percy Main Colliery on Tyneside. Brunel had been aware of this innovation, and had proposed cast iron linings for the Thames Tunnel, but the Company had rejected the proposal, and used a different section lined in brickwork. In 1824, just before the Thames Tunnel was started, Thomas Telford used temporary cast iron linings in the second Harecastle Tunnel. This used 16 segments bolted together as centering for the permanent lining of brickwork.

During the first half of the nineteenth century, engineers lodged several patents for different designs of tunnel-building shield, and gradually these evolved towards a practical system. In 1849, Samuel Dunn of Doncaster took out a patent for a tunnelling machine for use through soft sand and mud that was to utilize a cylindrical shield rammed forwards against the lining. In 1857, the French engineer Guibal designed a machine for sinking shafts through running wet sand, and in the 1860s, the Austro-Hungarian engineer and expert on sacred geometry Professor Rziha used a system of centres and face rams for driving various railway tunnels in central Europe. The perfect system, however, was invented in England. In 1862, Peter William Barlow was engaged on sinking the piers for Lambeth Bridge across the Thames in London, when the idea struck him that the methods being employed there could equally apply to horizontal tunnelling. In 1864, the same year that Parliament was alarmed at the prospect of a spate of cut-and-cover tunnelling, Barlow filed a patent for a tunnelling shield and its accompanying tunnel linings. "In constructing tunnels for railways", wrote Barlow, "particularly where the tunnels are to pass under rivers or under towns and places where the upper surface cannot without serious injury be broken up or interfered with, a cylinder of somewhat larger internal diameter than the external diameter of the intended tunnel is employed, such cylinder being by preference wrought iron or steel."

An attempt to build a tube railway under the Thames using a different system was made during the next year. Sir Charles Fox and T.W. Rammell designed a pneumatic-powered underground railway whose under-river section was to be four 235 ' lengths of cast iron tube ten feet in diameter, laid in a trench dredged in the river bed. In this trench, the tube was to be set upon piers formed from iron cylinders 21' in diameter, the top of the running tube resting beneath the Thames bed. In 1866, the trench was dredged, and two pillars nearest the Surrey shore were laid. A short brick-lined tunnel

191

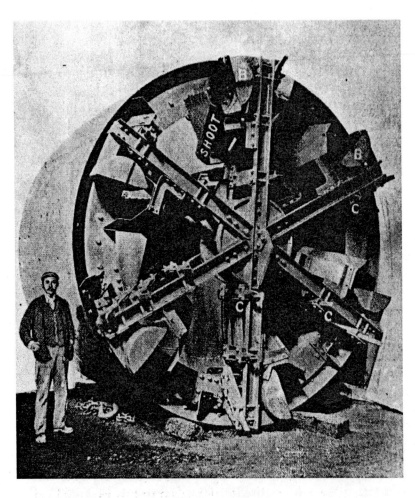

56. Price's electrically driven digging machine, used in 1899 for the tunnels of the Central London Railway. (Electric Traction Publications)

was built beneath College Street, and the first running tubes were fabricated. But the stock exchange crash of 1866 all but bankrupted the company, and work stopped. The piers in the river were removed for scrap, and the company wound up in 1882.

The Tower Subway

In 1868, undaunted by the failure of the pneumatic Waterloo and Whitehall Railway, Barlow put his proposals into action and floated a prospectus for the world's first segmentally-cast-iron-lined tube railway - the Tower Subway. This was to provide a river crossing from Vine Street, near Pickle Herring Wharf, on the south bank of the Thames, to Tower Hill on the north, a crossing further downstream than the traditional one at London Bridge (Tower Bridge did not exist then). The engineer of the tunnel was the South African, James Henry Greathead, perfector of the tunnelling shield. According to the great tube railway engineer Harley H. Dalrymple-Hay, Greathead's "invention of the tunnelling sheild named after him entitles him to be regarded as the practical author of the "Tubes of London". The Tower Subway was a single tube with an internal bore of 6 feet 7 3/4 inches. It was driven between two 10 foot diameter shafts, one 50 and the other 60 feet deep, and composed rings made of three segments 18 inches deep with a key in the crown of the tunnel. These segments were made from cast iron 7/8" thick with flanges of 2 1/8". The minimum cover of London Clay over the subway crown was 22 feet, and the overall length of the tunnel 1,350 feet. During construction, tunnelling proceeded at about 9 feet a day over three eight-hour shifts, and the overall cost of building the subway was £10,000.

Access to the tunnel was by way of steam-driven lifts which could carry 20 people. In the tunnel was a rail track of 30 inch gauge, upon which ran a truck pulled from end to end by a steel cable propelled by two 4 horsepower steam engines located at the foot of each shaft. When fully laden, the truck

193

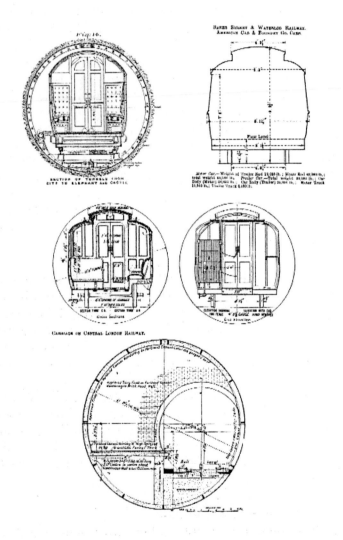

57. *Diagrams of early London undergraound railway carriages and tunnels. (Electric Traction Publications)*

carried 12 passengers. This railway, which was the only non-standard gauge passenger-carrying tube railway ever laid in London, was a failure, and the tunnel was soon converted into a footway, for the use of which pedestrians paid a toll. The lifts were replaced with spiral staircases when the railway was abandoned. The opening of Tower Bridge in 1895 led to the closure of the subway in 1896, when it was sold to the London Hydraulic Power Company for £3,000. This company laid two hydraulic mains through the Tower Subway to connect their new power station at Wapping to Rotherhithe and Bermondsey. The other LHPC mains crossed the river by Southwark, Waterloo and Vauxhall Bridges, and another hydraulic main was laid later in the tunnels of the City and South London Railway. The Tower Subway changed ownership again, when, after the abandonment of London's hydraulic power system in 1977, the Mercury Telecommunications company acquired the tunnel for use with fibre optic telecommunications cables.

The next tube railway, even less successful than the Tower Subway was built in New York in 1870, for the abortive Broadway Pneumatic Railway. It was a cast-iron tube 8 feet in diameter. Another short section of tube was built subsequently in Cincinnati. In England, the North and South Woolwich Subway project of 1876 was to use shields and cast-iron linings, but was abandoned by the contractors, owing to difficulties elsewhere. When commenced by T.A. Walker, who did not believe in the shield method of tunnelling, the work failed before long. Most subsequent tunnelling of tube railways in London has used a shield. The Greathead Shield or Rotary Shield were adopted for the earliest electrically-powered deep underground railways.

The Underground Mail

The origin of deep tube railways beneath the streets lies in Victorian experiments intended to overcome postal delays occasioned by traffic congestion. In 1853, J. Latimer Clark

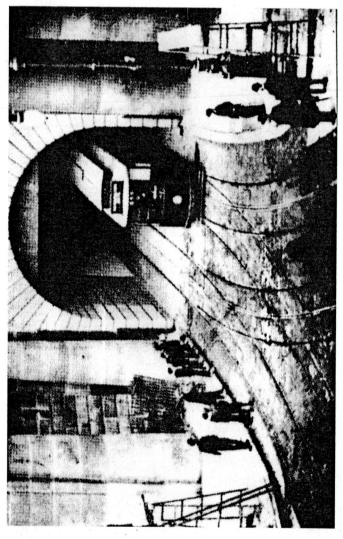

58. A single-decker tram of the London County Council on test, late in 1905. It is seen emerging from the south protal of the newly-constructed Kingsway Tramway Subway in central London, as illustrated on a contemporary postcard. (Electric Traction Publications)

laid a 1¹/₂" diameter tube the 625 feet between the offices of The Electrical and International Telegraph Company in Telegraph Street and the London Stock Exchange. Urgent messages were transmitted in small felt bags, blown through the tube by air from a compressor rated at six horsepower.

In 1855, officials of the General Post Office (GPO) made a report about the system, but rejected its adoption on the grounds that pipes at least 15 inches across would be needed to transport mails. But later, it seems that the value of underground transport was recognized, and the GPO laid many miles of 1 ¹/₂ in. lead pipe between post offices all over the Metropolis. By 1886, there were 94 lines in operation under London, totalling 34 ¹/₂ miles. Tubes were laid also in Dublin, Birmingham, Glasgow, Liverpool, Manchester and Newcastle-upon-Tyne: 129 lines with an aggregate mileage of 451/2, carrying 51,478 messages a day.

Although Latimer Clark's tubes were of small size, larger tubes figured in early experiments. In 1857, T.W. Rammell published a book titled *A New Plan For Street Railways*. In it, he proposed a network of subterranean mail tubes. On August 13 1859, The Pneumatic Dispatch Company obtained an Act of Parliament to lay tubes in the area of the Metropolitan Board of Works. An experimental tunnel was constructed at the Soho Works in Birmingham, and in 1861, it was exhibited at Battersea Fields in London. Inside the tube, which measured 30 by 33 inches, was an integrally-cast two-foot-gauge rail track. The vehicles that ran inside were fitted with vulcanized rubber flaps that made an airtight seal.

The experiment was judged successful, so a 30 inch tube, a third of a mile long line was built beneath the London streets. It linked the Number 1 arrival platform at Euston station with the North Western District post office in Eversholt St. Tests began on January 15 1863, five days after the opening of the first underground railway in the world, the steam-

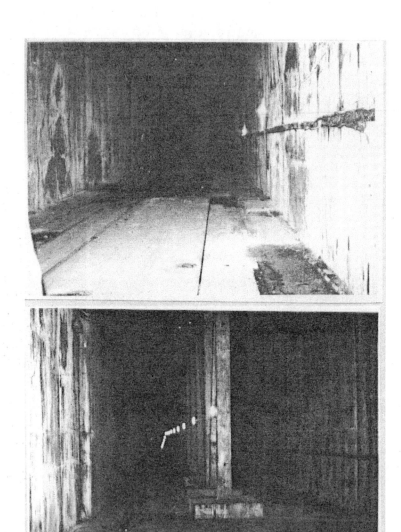

powered Metropolitan Railway. On February 20, the line was opened to traffic. Thirteen runs a day were the norm. Later, another line, 1 $^1/_2$ miles long, was built. Its route was Euston - Drummond Street - Hampstead Road. - Tottenham Court Road. - Broad Street Saint Giles' - to the company head-quarters at 245 High Holborn. The tunnel was 4 ft 6 in width by 4 ft high. It was constructed partly in cast-iron tube and partly in brick. Work began on September 23, 1863, and vehicles began operation October 10, 1865. The journey time was fast - only five minutes from end to end.

A third line was planned from Holborn to the GPO at Aldersgate and Pickfords' depot in Gresham St. Work began, but the collapse of Overend and Gurney's Bank in the 1866 Black Friday stock market crash led to the cessation of working from September 23 that year. By 1868, new funds had been secured to continue the work, and the extension began from Hatton Garden to the Old Post Office buildings in Cheapside - 1658 yards from Holborn and 4738 yards from Euston. This line opened for one-way traffic (cars being returned empty) on December 1, 1873. Transit of the line from end to end took only 17 minutes, but the line proved virtually inoperable and was abandoned on October 31 1874. The tubes then lay derelict, but between 1895 and 1896 were examined

Opposite: 59. Two views inside the abandoned tram subway under Kingsway, central London: above, the tunnel south of Holborn Station, showing tram track still in place. The slot is the 'conduit' for the undergroud power collection used by trams in central London. Below: the tunnel near Aldwych, showing the supports for the exit ramp of the Strand Underpass (1964) that occupies the southern end of the former tram tunnel, which was in service from 1905 until 1952. (both Nigel Pennick)

by the Post Office consulting engineer, George Threlfall, with a view to conversion to electric traction. Threlfall and some board members of the now-defunct owning company formed the London Despatch Company Ltd. in May 1899. The company made some repairs to the tube, but the Post Office was not interested, and refurbishment ceased in 1902. In 1905, the London Despatch Company was wound up.

After that, the tunnels took the interest of other private utilities. Opportunistically, various gas and electric companies began to use the tunnels, which appeared to have no owner and were unregulated. On December 20, 1928, the result of this unregulation was an enormous gas explosion in the tunnel beneath High Holborn. It blew up almost half a mile of road. In 1930, during a survey, Post Office engineers rediscovered four of the original vehicles abandoned in the tunnel. They were taken out and scrapped. In the same year, more cars (but of the narrower, earlier, line) were found under Eversholt Street, and three were preserved. One was sent to Bruce Castle Museum in Tottenham, another went to the museum in Kingston-upon-Hull. It was destroyed when the museum was bombed in World War II. A third was sent to the Museum of London. To-day, the ecologically sound and technically practical idea of sending items underground by pneumatic power is ignored, and motorcycle couriers pollute the streets.

Most of these tunnels still exist beneath the streets of London. Part of the Holborn tunnel was destroyed in 1905 during construction of the Kingsway Tramway Subway and later, further parts were destroyed in the gas explosion of 1928 and the reconstruction of Chancery Lane and St Paul's tube stations (1932-4 & 1935-9 respectively). The reconstruction of Euston mainline station in 1963 destroyed further sections.

Chapter Twelve

The Urban Folklore of the London Underground

It would be strange if a major installation of some antiquity used by millions of people every day did not generate many misconceptions about it, and produce its own internal lore. Most of the lore detailed here has been received directly by the author from various Cockney sources. Obviously, it must be incomplete, as new stories are forever emerging.

Urban legends about tube lines may be divided into those concerning construction; those concerning operation; and those concerning other incidents. There is one curious 'coincidence' to begin with: the 'circle and bar' motif used since the early part of the century to denote the Underground (written with upper case terminal 'D'), and subsequently extended to the rest of London Transport, is one old alchemical symbol for earth!

Construction

There is an archetypal folk-tale told of various tunnels. Workmen were digging at the face of the tunnel, when a ghastly apparition manifested itself. They flung down their picks and shovels and fled, swearing that never again would they work there. This tale is told to explain the abandonment of the extension of the Great Northern and City Railway from Moorgate to Lothbury in 1904. The tunnelling shield used in digging the tunnels is said to be left embedded in the London

201

Clay to this day. The tale attaches also to the Victoria Line at Pimlico (built in the early 1970s), and to tunnels under a nuclear power station on Anglesey.

A corollary of these tales is that the workmen were Irish, adding to the hearer's expectations of superstitious terror. In the 1960s, the construction of the Victoria Line led to the creation of one of Euan MacColl's most evocative folksongs, *The Tunnel Tigers* commemorating the Irish navvies working beneath the city streets far from the sun and the light of day. Written in 1966, it used the traditional Wexford tune, *Willie Taylor*, it was recorded by The Johnstons and broadcast in a BBC television documentary about the new tube line, "driving a tunnel through the London Clay".

Presumably, the basis of these tales (which may exist all over the world) comes from the belief that the spirits of the Earth, disturbed by the tunnellers, are forced to expel the intruders. An alternative explanation, possible in hard rock but unlikely in the London Clay, is the triggering of an electrostatic phenomenon. This theme was taken by the 1960s television play *Quatermass and the Pit,* an early 'ancient astronauts' motif which linked poltergeists, ghostly apparitions, tube railway construction and prehistoric spacecraft.

Linked to the supposed apparitions seen by Irish navvies are the explanations for 'deviations' in the apparently 'obvious' course of tube lines. These stories are a variant of Urban Architecture Lore, which tells of buildings being accidentally constructed the wrong way round because of the misreading of plans. Sharp curves on tube lines, such as that on the Piccadilly by the Brompton Oratory, between the abandoned Brompton Road station and South Kensington, are attributed to the engineering necessity to avoid 'plague pits'. At South Kensington, the westbound line is 78 feet deep, and the eastbound 60 feet, far below any supposed 'plague pit'. The reason for this deviation is in this section of the line's genesis as part of the District Deep Level express tube. However, these reasons are not easy to grasp, or easily found out about, and so a folkloristic explanation has evolved in the last 80 years. I have heard the same story connected with the curve in the Bakerloo line between Regent's Park and Baker Street, and also the curve between St Pauls and Bank stations on the Central Line. And of course, the Pimlico apparition was attributable to a 'plague pit'.

Another Urban Architecture-type tale tells of how the junction at Holborn on the Piccadilly Line was meant to join up the twin tubes of the 'main line' to the twin tubes of the branch to Aldwych, but the drawing office got it wrong, and lined up the tunnels on the same level, making it impossible to, operate the branch line integrally with the rest of the line. Finally, this led to its closure in the 1990s.

Operational Folklore

Underground train operations are taken for granted by passengers, who rarely give a second thought to them except when something untoward occurs. People are always apprehensive of being lost, especially below ground. One such legend is of a train making an unscheduled stop at an abandoned station. Someone, or a number of people, mistakenly get out, thinking it to be their stop. Then they are trapped there for days before escaping. But as abandoned stations are poorly lit or unlit, and the doors of deep-level trains are operated by a button pressed by the guard, or by the driver on one-man trains, even if a train should stop at one of these abandoned stations, then the doors would not open.

The worst tube accident yet, which took place on February 28, 1975 is still unexplained. The 8.37 a.m. six-carriage train from Drayton Park entered the terminal Platform 9 at Moorgate and accelerated into the dead-end of the tunnel constructed for the Lothbury extension. 41 passengers and the driver died and 74 were injured. At the inquest, eye-witnesses told of how the driver was seemingly transfixed at the controls, but as the cab was smashed almost flat (10 cm deep) by the impact, and it took a long time digging out the mangled wreckage, it was impossible to do a post-mortem on the driver's remains. Tube trains have a safety device known as the 'dead man's handle', which must be depressed by the driver at all times. If it is released, for example, if the driver has a heart attack, then the brakes are applied. This did not happen at the Moorgate accident, and so it was assumed that the driver had not had a seizure. Urban lore connects the driver's 'transfixion' with the Lothbury extension 'apparition' of 1904, perhaps a re-manifestation. The best known tube apparition is at Covent Garden station on the Piccadilly Line, at over a hundred feet below the surface, the deepest on the line. Here, a ghost of a man, said to be the actor William Terriss, who killed himself, mounts the spiral emergency staircase, but vanishes before he reaches the top.

'Lost trains', Odd Happenings and Other Incidents

An experimental pneumatically-powered Victorian tube line in the grounds of Crystal Palace may have given rise to another genre of tube legends. When the line was abandoned, and the car or train was buried with it, this knowledge may have been subtly altered by oral transmission into the 'lost train' mythos. This piece of urban folklore states that somewhere under London is a train which was walled-up full of dead passengers. The stories surrounding this explain it by stating that there was some unavoidable reason for not removing the dead passengers - unexploded bombs, etc. - or that they were walled up alive. Perhaps this motif comes from a combination of the Balham bomb disaster during the Blitz, and one of the Rev. W. Awdry's stories of Thomas The Tank Engine and Friends, where a locomotive is walled up in a tunnel as a punishment for his intransigence. In 1978, the *London Evening News* reported that a 19 year-old woman named Pamela Goodsall had fallen into the remains of the Crystal Palace tunnel.

The commercial pneumatic operation of the two mail lines in central London, although used for mail, occasional VIP passengers were carried for fun, and lore tells of a Victorian lady in Crinoline dress who leant too near the tunnel entrance, fell in and was blown from one end of the line to the other. The fact that Crinolines had been superseded by bustle dresses by then does not detract from the story. On December 20, 1928 half a mile of Holborn street was blown out by a gas exposion in the by-now abandoned tunnel, occasioned by a workmen lighting a last fatal cigarette.

'Lost Trains', or at least mail cars, were discovered beneath Cheapside in 1930 by Post Office engineers as a result of the work occasioned by the explosion. One was in Hull Museum until destroyed in World War II, whilst another went to Bruce Castle Museum, Tottenham, and a third to the Museum of London. 'Lost Train' lore is, of course, more baroque than this, including a train blown apart in the war and filled in with concrete (complete with bodies!) at Bethnal Green or King's Cross or the abandoned station of British Museum (take your pick). Bethnal Green tube station was not opened to trains until 1946, a year after the end of the war, but during the war saw a major disaster when panicking shelterers cascaded down an escalator, crushing many to death. Perhaps this is the garbled origin of the 'Lost Train' tale there. Other 'lost train' principles may relate to the train enthusiasts' Cold War rumour concerning old locomotives and rolling stock allegedly stashed away for use after World War III (presumably by the Soviet Army of Occupation!). The recent restoration to service of '1938' tube trains brought back temporarily from the scrapyard must give rise to more tales of this sort.

The reasons for building whole underground rail installations often owe a lot to urban folklore. It is said that the Baker

Street and Waterloo Railway was first thought of as a way for Westminster businessmen to get to see the last overs at Lord's cricket ground after work. As far as I am aware, the motif of the line built to avoid the untoward effects of military pomp and circumstance is unknown in London. However, Germany affords such instances. It is said that the former 4-track tram subway beneath the avenue called Unter Den Linden in Berlin was installed because the Kaiser's army held so many daily parades that the only way to run the trams on time was to put them beneath the road. This tunnel was destroyed in World War II. A similar tale was told of the Nuremberg tram subway which was built under Nazi rule, this time to avoid the endless parades of the Party.

Human Terror on the Tube

Aberrant human behaviour on the Underground can be observed at all times, from the results of spray-can-wielding youth to rampaging football hooligans and 'steaming' gangs of robbers. The motif of 'the maniac on the platform' first noted by Michael Goss, is an important one in urban paranoia. According to this story, the Maniac stands on crowded platforms, and, just as a train is entering the station, pushes a young woman in front of it. Naturally, the police have suppressed publicity of these events to avoid 'carbon copy crime'. Of course, the perpetrator of these supposed crimes is still at large...

The blues musician Graham Bond of the group called *Magick,* whose last records dealt with the occult traditions of the Order of the Golden Dawn and the Matter of Britain, died beneath an underground train at Finsbury Park station in 1973. It was said that he fell beneath an incoming train, being horribly mutilated, but that the Egyptian amulet that he was wearing was undamaged.

Chapter Thirteen

Some More British Subterranea

Essex and East Anglia

Once described as 'the most haunted house in England', Borley Rectory in Essex has a reputation which has survived its destruction by fire in 1939. The psychical phenomena so long associated with the Rectory have now transferred themselves to the nearby church, and because of this research has continued there.

For a long time the Rectory was the site of a legendary tunnel which in 1924 was found to be a genuine folk memory. In that year a Mr Farrance was repairing a well for the rector when a tunnel was encountered. Walled up without further investigation, it was re-discovered during sewer works in 1957. Running from the Rectory to the Church, it is brick-lined tunnel whose use is unknown: it cannot have been a sewer because changes in gradient within the tunnel would prevent free drainage. It remains a mystery to this day.

The Anstey tunnel in Hertfordshire has been mentioned in Chapter 7 in connection with the legend of Blind George, the resident fiddler of the Chequers Inn. Unlike many subterranea, parts of this tunnel have been explored. It is said to run from Cave Gate to the moat at Anstey Castle a mile distant. All that remains of the castle now is a moated mount, but in this moat is a most interesting feature discovered

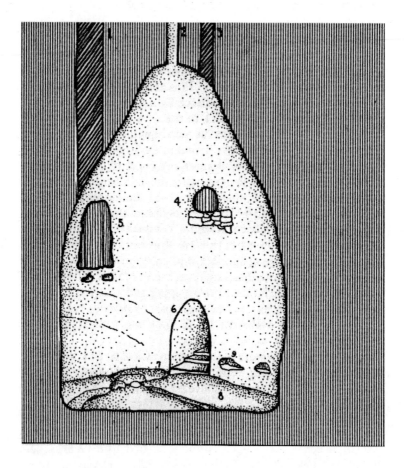

60. The Royston Cave, section: 1. Original entrance, now sealed; 2. Present ventilation shaft; 3. Old shaft, now sealed; 4,5 Entrances of shafts; 6. Present entrance; 7. 'The Grave' aperture in floor; 8. Floor; 9. Ritual niches. (Nigel Pennick)

during a drought in about 1862. One of the workmen employed to clean the moat during the drought, a Thomas Martin, remembered as an old man in 1902 having encountered a pair of iron gates embedded in the mud of the moat. Martin cleaned them, but was told that on no account should they be opened, as the 'government' had refused the farmer's request to find out where they led.

These gates were last seen in 1921 when the moat was again cleaned, but the summer was not so dry as 1862, and the water level rose again quickly and the gates were submerged. Local tradition asserts that these gates were the exit of the tunnel whose entrance lies a mile away at Cave Gate where the drama of Blind George is set. Locally it is said that in the fields at several places on the line between Cave Gate and Anstey not only does the wheat fail to grow as well as elsewhere, but that during the winter the snow at those points melts earlier. Thomas Martin remarked in 1902 that there were certain places in the fields where stones and earth had been heard to fall below ground from time to time. Such an interesting tunnel would obviously repay further investigation and at the time of writing preliminary investigations have begun on the Anstey moat.

Of all British subterranea, the strange cave at Royston in Hertfordshire is the most enigmatic. In August 1742, workmen were erecting a new bench in the Butter Market at Royston, when one of them noticed a millstone embedded in the ground. Lifting it up, to his amazement he discovered a shaft leading downwards into the chalk. Excited by the find, the workmen lowered first a boy, then a thin man, into the cavity, which turned out to be a bell-shaped structure more than half filled with earth.

News of the find spread rapidly round the small market town and there was no shortage of enthusiastic people willing to dig out the earth in the hope of finding buried treasure. Working

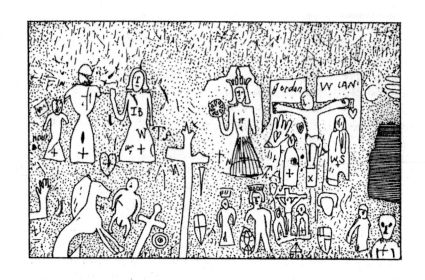

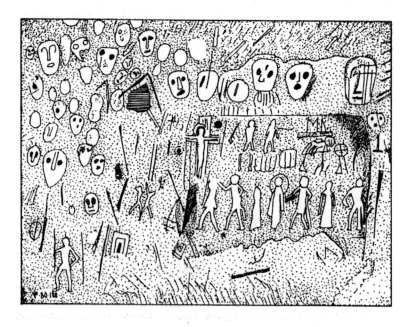

61. Carvings at the Royston Cave (upper) compared with the Burgstein (lower). (Nigel Pennick)

210

at night to avoid the crowds of sightseers, workmen soon removed several cartloads of soil from the cave. Scientific archaeology was then unknown, and whatever was found in the soil deposits - a few bones and some fragments of pottery - were discarded as worthless. However, the diggers revealed a series of carvings the like of which cannot be seen anywhere else this side of the Czech Republic.

Naturally such a remarkable find came to the notice of eminent antiquaries who flocked from far and wide to examine the cave. William Stukeley visited the site and in 1744 wrote a treatise titled *Origines Roystoniae* in which he forwarded theories about the cave. The reverend Charles Parkin, rector of Oxburgh, Norfolk, begged to differ, and attempted to refute Stukeley's ideas in a pamphlet of his own. At that time the theory emerged that the cave had been a hermitage connected in some way with the shadowy figure of Lady Roisia de Vere, legendary foundress of Royston. Stukeley thought the carvings depicted scenes from her family history and that the cave was an oratory or chantry for the family, whilst Parkin thought that it was nothing more than a hermitage.

In 1790, during an exceptionally hard winter, a local contractor employed his men to cut a new passage to the cave as a kind of early unemployment relief programme. This entrance is in use now, for the original entrance was from above by a narrow and precarious shaft. Visitors continued to flock to the cave, and in 1852 Joseph Beldam published the results of his own researches. Having dug up into the remaining earth of the floor and found fragments of bone, iron, wood, leather and some ' decorative stones', he claimed that the cave had formerly been a Romano-British shaft, later modified as a Roman *columbarium* or shaft-grave, then finally modified as a Christian oratory. Sylvia Beamon believes that the cave was connected with the heretical Knights Templar who between 1199 and 1254 had a weekly market stall as

211

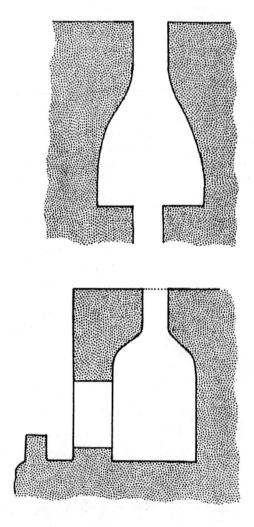

62. *The aberrant form of well-construction at Warwick is echoed by the strange bottle-shaped cave at the Burgstein, Ceska Lipa, Czech Republic. (Nigel Pennick)*

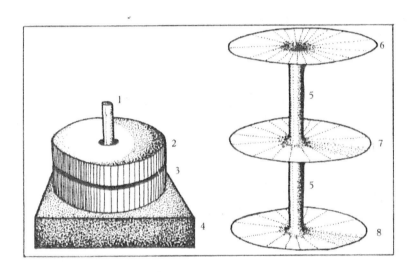

*63. Cosmological symbolism of the world axis as a mill: (1)
The axle-tree; (2) the moving upper stone symbolic of the
heavens; (3) the stationary lower stone symbolises the earth; (4)
the ground is the underworld into which the axle-tree
penetrates. paralleling the cosmic concept of (5) the world tree,
which links (6) the heavenly upperworld with (7) the earthly
middleworld with (8) the incorporeal underworld. (Nigel
Pennick)*

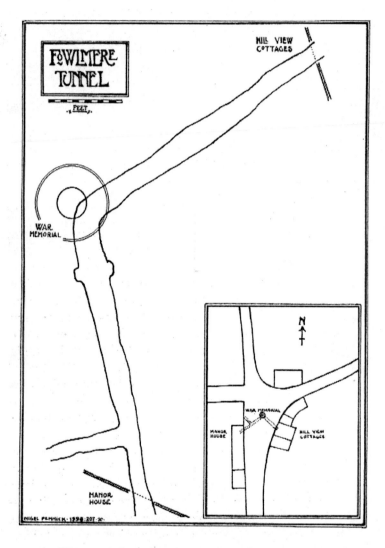

64. *The tunnel under the road in the village centre at Fowlmere, Cambridgeshire, linking the Old Manor House and Hill View Cottages. (Nigel Pennick, after Subterranea Britannica (1974) with author's own survey)*

Royston and travelled there from the headquarters at Baldock nine miles to the west. Excavations by Miss Donal demonstrated that there could have been at one time a floor dividing the cave into an upper and a lower storey, and Sylvia Beamon believes that the upper part could have been a store for Templar wares whilst the lower floor was a chapel for their peculiar devotions.

The most notable feature of the Royston Cave is the profusion of carvings which cover the walls. Although in recent years vibration from heavy traffic has destroyed several of the carvings, the majority still survive. Christian saints and crucifixion scenes intermingle with more ancient Pagan themes: human heads, a Sheela-na-Gig, a horse, sunwheels and holds holding hearts. Sylvia Beamon has noted the similarity of many of these carvings with graffiti made by the Knights Templar when incarcerated in the Tour du Coudray at Chinon in France, and similar carvings were described by the German researcher E. Gebauer in the ancient mysteries journal *Germanien* in 1935. Gebauer described the strange bottle-shaped cave in the *Burgstein*, a weird outcrop of rock by the village of Svojka near Ceska Lipa in the Czech Republic. The cave itself is a striking parallel with that at Royston, of which Gebauer makes no mention, though its dimensions are slightly smaller twenty-one feet deep by ten feet wide as compared with the English cave at twenty-nine by eighteen.

Bottle-shaped subterranea are uncommon, but for some as yet undetermined reason they seem to have been popular in Warwick. In 1958, a bottle-shaped pit was found in Jury Street, Warwick, and ten years later a second such pit was found under premises in Brook Street, containing the skeletons of cats and chickens as well as the usual debris. A bottle-shaped well was excavated in that city in Swan Street in 1972, but nothing has been suggested to account for this unusual form, and none of the subterranea there had any carvings. The Ceska Lipa cave has carved figures which are remarkably similar to those which cover the walls of the Royston Cave, including a crucifix, various human figures bearing arms, crosses, runes, sunwheels and detached human heads. Several of the carvings at Royston have a Pagan flavour to - the Sheela-na-Gig is the most blatant - and even the Christian saints are those whose pagan origin is plain to see. One of the most prominent figures is that of a crowned woman holding aloft an eight-spoked wheel. Naturally, she is seen as St Catherine with her instrument of martyrdom. But the Queen of the Underworld, Persephone, was also depicted in this way on the holy vessels of the Orphic religion: the hanging wheel on a series of Orphic Greek vases depicting the underworld now in the Naples Museum is an allusion to a little known Orphic hymn:

I have flown out of the sorrowful weary circle,
I have passed with swift feet to the diadem desired,
I have sunk beneath the bosom of the Mistress, the Queen of the Underworld,
And now I come as a supplicant to Holy Persephone.

The crowned woman at Royston is surely Queen of the Underworld, whether or not the carver knew it. The carving of St Christopher, sporting an uncharacteristic phallus in his guise as a Christianized Hermes, is another indicator of the connection with hermits and wayfarers, but also the aspect of travelling across the rivers of the underworld, for the geomantic position of the Royston Cave is absolutely correct for an entrance to the underworld. Situated at the crossing-point of two major Roman routes, the Icknield Way and Ermine Street, the cave echoes ancient cosmology, for the sacred shaft at the crossroads was a fundamental part of gemantic lore. The practice of making such shafts has come down to use from the Etruscans, whose geomancy was a precise art whose major function was the auspicious foundation of cities according to cosmological principles.

The fourfold division of the world known from many disparate cultures was the fundamental principle of Etruscan geomancy. At the centre of the two lines which divided the world was the central point now universally known by its Greek name of *omphalos*. The discovery of the local counterpart of this 'navel of the world' was the task of the Augur, who by divination marked the correct point for the centre of the new city. After fixing the north-south and east-west lines by celestial observation, the Augur took his staff of office, the *lituus*, a forerunner of the modern Christian Pastoral Staff carried by bishops, and with it solemnly marked out the two roads crossing at the *omphalos*. There, where the axes crossed, a deep shaft was dug. This was seen to connect the world of the living with the under- world of the dead. The top was sealed with stone slabs.

Such a cavern was called the *mundus,* the word also used for the vault of the heavens, of which it was a subterraneous reflection. According to the author Varro, the mundus was the gateway to the gods of the nether regions. When this had been constructed, then the rituals of boundary-making and the casting of lots for pieces of land in the new city could be carried out.

Royston is the only perfect geomantic site in Britain. At the intersection of two straight roads oriented to the cardinal directions was not only the cave, entry to the underworld, but a large mark-stone, later socketed for a standing cross. The stone is known as the Roy Stone, from which the town takes its name. Here we have a classic *omphalos,* with its three levels: the cave representing the deathly underworld; the crossroads representing the earthly middleworld; and the stone representing access to the spiritual upperworld. As if to ram home this symbolism, the original discoverers of the cave found that it had been sealed with a millstone. The millstone is here doubly symbolic for it was with a millstone set in grooves that the tombs of the Jews in ancient Palestine were

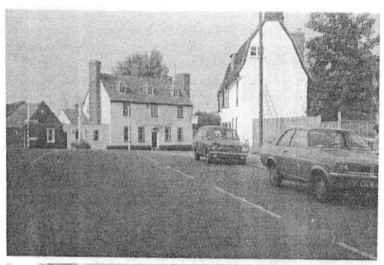

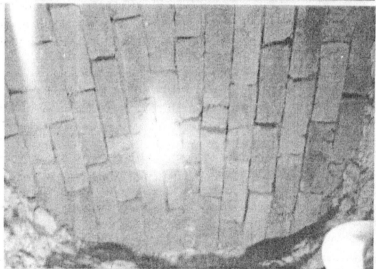

65. *Fowlmere, Cambridgeshire, England: Above, the tunnel runs beneath the street here, passing beneath the War Memorial (middle left). Below: Inside the Fowlmere Tunnel. This brickwork (1922) supports the War Memorial at the middle of the tunnel. (Nigel Pennick)*

sealed. The rolling away of the stone from the mouth of Christ's tomb records the use of such a millstone. In ancient northern Europe, millstones with their axle tree also symbolized the whole cosmic system: the upper stone rotating as the heavens; the lower stone stationary as the earth; the axletree linking the upper with the lower, set into the earth in a pit which represented the underworld.

Bury St Edmunds, Suffolk

Many ancient underground tunnels remain forgotten for years until a sudden collapse brings them forcibly into the glare of public scrutiny. In 1977, after a rainstorm, a large hole suddenly appeared in the street of a housing estate at Sudbury, Suffolk. Unfortunately for students of subterranea, this hole was filled in the very next day, and no exploration was attempted. In nearby Bury St Edmunds, a much longer tale revolves around a forgotten tunnel network - a tale without a happy ending.

In May 1955 a plumber named Percy Cook was called into 4 Willow Cottages, Bury St Edmunds, to unblock a lavatory. Lifting the cover of a manhole, he sent an assistant to pull the chain. On performing this mundane task, the floor literally opened up beneath his feet, and he fell fifty feet to the bottom of a cavity. He was finally rescued from the hole, and it was filled in. In 1959, the West Suffolk Hospital Management Board decided that a lot of land to the north of the Bury St Edmunds Hospital was surplus to requirements, and offered to sell it to the local authority. The Borough Surveyor, having heard rumours that the ground was unsafe, and in knowledge of the lavatory incident, advised the Housing and Parks Committee of the council not to purchase the land.

The area was finally auctioned, and in 1964 a local builder became its owner. Planning permission to erect a number of houses was granted by the council, and the ownership of the

land then passed to a developer who commenced construction
of terraces of split-level town houses.

The new development was given the name Jacqueline Close.
When an intending home buyer applied to the council for a
mortgage on one of the new properties, the council rejected his
application on the grounds that the area was reputed to be
undermined. On hearing of this serious possibility, the
developers commissioned two reports, one from a Cambridge
geologist, Dr C. L. Forbes, and the other from Rock Mechanics
Ltd., of Chelsea.

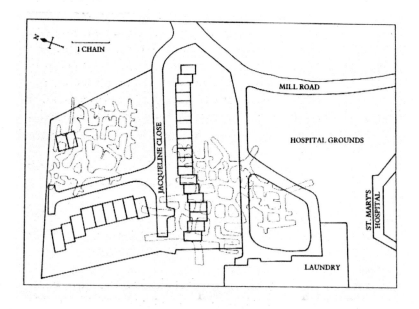

66. *Map of the abandoned chalk mine under Jacqueline Close,
Bury St Edmunds, Suffolk. (Nigel Pennick after Harry
Pearman)*

The Cambridge scientist visited the site and discovered that there was probably a chalk mine forty feet beneath the surface. Twenty foot borings by the geological consultants found nothing, and although their report inferred that as the land was solid to this depth and that it was sound enough to support houses, they denied responsibility if the estate's drainage was poorly sited. This is exactly what the drainage plan turned out to be; the soakaways had the effect of concentrating the area's rainwater onto specific points on the tunnels' roofs.

Inevitably, the collapses began. In July 1967, a twenty-seven foot deep hole appeared. Ready-mixed concrete was brought in and the hole was filled. In December of that year another drain caved in and concrete was again poured in. A year later, after talks about a new drainage system had proved fruitless, a massive fall of rain caused a major cave-in. The front path, patio and a large part of the foundations of number 9 Jacqueline Close slipped into a shaft twenty feet wide by thirty feet deep. The council declared the site unsafe, and many residents left. Members of the Chelsea Speleological Society, a much respected cave exploration club, were called in to explore the workings.

A large chalk mine with walls so fragile that one touch would cause a fall appeared in the speleologists' torch-beams. A survey was instituted and it soon became clear that not only was the Close completely undermined by old workings, but that the northern section of the adjoining hospital also had unsafe tunnels beneath it.

Local enquiries finally revealed that during the nineteenth century there had been subterranean extensions to an open chalk quarry, known as Bullen's Lime Kiln on the 25" Ordnance Survey Map. One old resident remembered sending beer in a basket down a shaft to refresh the miners working below.

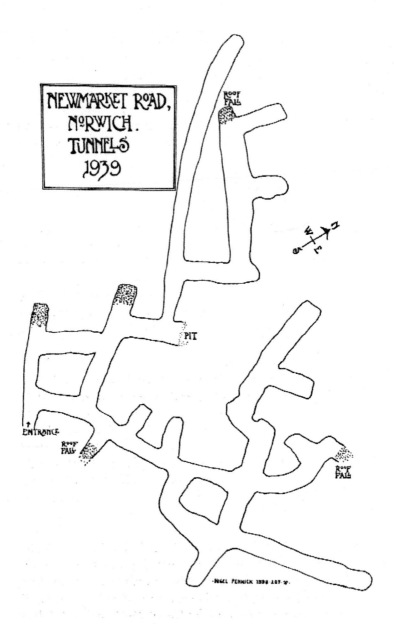

67. Tunnels in the vicinity of Newmarket Road, Norwich, Norfolk, England, as surveyed in 1939. (Nigel Pennick)

The portion of the mine beneath the hospitals was filled almost immediately with fly ash, the standard substance used to dispose of old mines and deneholes. The residents, lacking the assistance of public moneys, could not afford such a course of action. Some of the houses were then just abandoned, and have fallen derelict or proved attractive to squatters and vandals, a salutary lesson to those who would ignore local lore.

Grimes Graves

The extraction of flint can safely be termed the oldest industry of Britain. It is still practised at Brandon only three miles away from the earliest mines at Grimes Graves. In an area of only sixteen and a half acres, there are no fewer than 366 known flint mines dating from as early as 2700 B.C. They are of two distinct types: the simpler were bell-pits of the type used 4000 years later in medieval England; and deep shafts with radiating galleries.

In one of these galleries, a 'votive shrine' was found. The section of the mine, for geological reasons, had failed to provide flint of an acceptable quality, and it was found to contain a pile of flints covered with antler-picks. On a ledge overlooking this offering was a chalk figurine of a pregnant woman, and in the entrance to a nearby gallery, the male principle was recognized in the form of chalk balls and a phallus. Recently, these figures have been exposed as fakes, placed there in the 1930s.

The religious meaning of such a shrine, if genuine, would be clear at Grimes Graves, as are the carvings in the Royston Cave. But little is known of the carvings at Eastry, Chislehurst and Boleigh. What is certain is that miners of all ages who probed the dangerous depths of Mother Earth felt a need for some protection from the likelihood of death or serious injury befalling them.

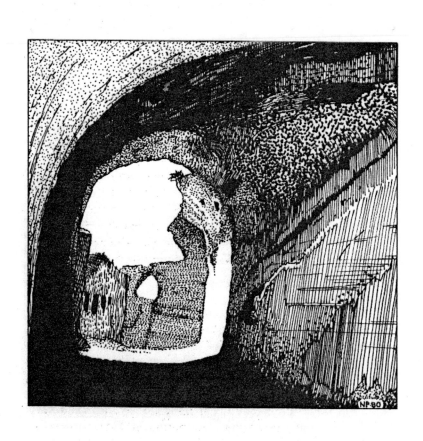

68. Mortimer's Hole, Nottingham Castle Rock. (Nigel Pennick)

Nottingham

In the ninth century a Welsh monk named Asser wrote what is now the earliest reference to the city of Nottingham. In his *The Life of King Alfred* he relates that the town was called in the British language (Welsh) 'Tigguocobaucc', which means 'the house of caves'. Even at that period the inhabitants had realized that the soft Bunter Sandstone which underlies the area and outcrops as the Castle Rock is an ideal medium in which to excavate caves and cellars.

The present name of the city is a translation of Tigguocobaucc from Welsh into Anglo-Saxon, for *snodenge* means caves and *ham* a house. The town became known as Snodengeham which has become corrupted into the modern Nottingham.

Many people lived in cave dwellings cut into the side of the cliffs which were formed by two sandstone outcrops in the city - the Castle Rock and the Lace Market district. The logical extension of these rock-cut dwellings was to construct a house on the front, and soon places not built against cliff faces had underground rooms burrowed beneath the floors. Many of these vast cellar complexes still exist today despite wholesale filling-in during redevelopment, over a hundred having been charted.

The Castle Rock is perforated by many holes, apertures and tunnels, the best known and most romantic of which is Mortimer's Hole. A passage 107 yards long, the name of this tunnel recalls the sad tale of Roger Mortimer, Earl of March, who in 1327 was instrumental in murdering King Edward II, after which he acted as Regent of England with the assistance of the late king's widow, Queen Isabella. In 1330, during a progress through the realm, Mortimer held a Parliament at Nottingham, and whilst at the castle he was arrested in the Queen's apartments on the order of Edward III. The deputy constable of the castle entered, unknown to Mortimer, by way of the secret passage through which the hapless Regent was removed a prisoner to London and thence to the scaffold at Tyburn.

Of this and other caves in the Castle Rock the geographer John Speede wrote in 1610:

'Many strange Vaults hewed out of the rocks in this Towne are seene, and those under the Castle of an especiall note, one for the story of Christ and His Passion engraven in the Walls, cut by the Hand of David, the second King of Scots, whilst he was therein detained prisoner; Another therein Lord Mortimer was surprised in the Non-age of King Edward III, since bearing the name of Mortimer's Hold; these have their Staires and severall Roomes made artificiallie even out of the Rocks: as also that Hill are dwelling Houses with winding Staires, Windows, Chimneies and Roome above Roome wrought all out of the solid Rock.'

Various of the underground passages and apertures in Castle Rock have yet to be fully explored, like many of the other holes burrowed under the city streets. Many underground structures in Nottingham were no more than the cellars found under most towns, but owing to the favourable terrain they tended to be deeper and more complex than those in places with a less favourable geology. Many of them were simply storage of one kind or another; most of the old inns of the city had extensive rock-cut cellars for the storage of beers and liquors. Those at the Salutation Inn can still be seen, complete with channels and holes which mark the course of the pipes leading from the beer pumps to the barrels of ale stored deep beneath the ground.

In his book *The History of Nottinghamshire,* published in 1751, Charles Deering recounted the fame of Nottingham's ale. This indisputable superiority was because the inns possessed the 'best, coolest and deepest rock cellars to store their liquor in, many being twenty, twenty-four to thirty-six

226

steps down, nay, in some places there are cellars within cellars, deeper and deeper in the rock'.

In addition to storing beer, several subterranean places served as factories for malt. Redevelopment in Castle Gate exposed a set of caves with a malt kiln and a cave identified as a store for malt or barley still exists in the Bridlesmith Gate complex, and in addition to the manufacture and storage of ale underground, it is still possible to drink it in two rock-cut bars of the fine public house *The Trip To Jerusalem*, which claims to be the oldest in England. Clandestine drinking took place during the eighteenth century in the notorious 'drinking cellars', and other subterranea served as gambling dens or cock-fighting pits.'Underground' activities in Nottingham were literally underground.

During the last century, a company was formed to construct a catacomb system for the burial of Nottingham's dead. At the top of the hill on Mansfield Road, the cemetery company started the Rock Cemetery, a series of tunnels large enough for a horse-drawn hearse to be driven inside. The company went bankrupt before the catacombs were completed, and they were abandoned without a single burial taking place in them.

Half a mile to the north of the medieval city, to the west of the Mansfield Road, were sand mines. It was the custom of Nottingham housewives to buy a pennyworth of sand to spread on the floor of the house in place of the traditional rushes, and the sale of sand doubtless proved profitable for those who were excavating cellars beneath their properties. The mine under Peel Street off the Mansfield Road was constructed at some time during the eighteenth century and is still accessible to the public. At the height of its production, so much sand was being excavated that a narrow-gauge railway worked by horse traction was installed, for the building trade in Nottingham depended heavily on this

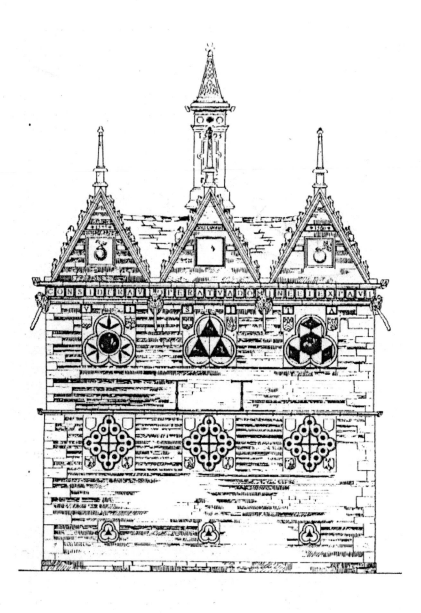

69. *The Triangular Lodge at Rushdon in Northamptonshire,
England, south-west elevation. (Nideck)*

source. After a miner was killed, however, the Corporation in 1806 had part of the mine blown up with gun- powder, and the trade declined.

During World War II, underground Nottingham was a warren of air-raid shelters. During the Munich Crisis a start had been made on a vast shelter to house the entire population of the city in the event of air raids, but it was never opened to the public. Some of the larger factories burrowed into the rock to make shelters for their workers, and the famous caves and cellars were pressed to a new use. In more recent times, the caves have served as mushroom farms, social clubs, a research centre for the investigation of cosmic rays and even as a rifle range. As redevelopment continues in the city, more and more subterranea will come to light, and the Nottingham Historical Arts Association is doing sterling work in recording and preserving the caves as they are discovered. They have managed to save the systems at Drury Hill (beneath the Broad Marsh shopping centre) and Bridlesmith Gate, which they open to the public. They are well worth a visit.

The Triangular Lodge, Rushton, Northants

The Rushton triangular lodge is one of the great geomantic buildings of the English Renaissance. A mystical tribute to the Holy Trinity, the lodge was designed by the devout Roman Catholic Sir Thomas Tresham, who made everything triangular or numbered in threes.

A measured survey of this singular piece of devotional architecture has revealed that there is an unaccounted space behind the fireplace on the top floor, a discovery which has given rise to the typical legends. Whatever the purpose of this secret hiding-place, there is also a tunnel legend associated with the lodge which asserts that a passage connects it with the main building of the Hall. Some time ago, during the reconstruction of the drains, a stone slab with a ring was

229

actually discovered in the cellar. On lifting the stone, a space below was revealed, but it was filled in with rocks and left unexamined.

The legend of the Rushton tunnel is typical. In the latter part of the eighteenth century, the owner of the estate, Lord Robert Cullen, found the secret passage but was too afraid to enter it. He offered a reward of £50 to anyone who would explore the tunnel for him, and the offer was taken up by the obligatory local fiddler, who took the £50 and gave it to his wife before entering the passage. Illuminated by a candle on his hat in the manner of the miners of the period, and playing the folk air *Moll in the Wad,* the brave fiddler strode forward underground. Suddenly, the music stopped, and he was never heard ofagain. His friends went to look for him, but all they found was his hat beside a deep pit, down which, it was assumed, the fiddler had fallen to his doom.

The story ends in farce. Two years after the event, the wife received a letter from the fiddler, who had supposedly fallen right through the world to Australia. The locals clubbed together to pay her fare to join him, and she left the village with a tidy sum. If true, the tale records a monumental confidence trick played upon the simple folk of Rushton.

Tresham may have indeed constructed an escape tunnel from the Lodge, as his Catholic faith was a treasonable offence at the time. The likelihood is increased by a similar tunnel at his other geomantic building, the Lyveden New Building near Oundle, which was a cruciform structure intended as another devotional exercise in stone, but never completed owing to its owner's death. Granville Squires in his book *Secret Hiding Places* quotes the eminent authority on Renaissance architecture J. A. Gotch, who discovered the remains of a passage at the south entrance. It led south-westerly towards the woods, but, like so many fascinating tunnels, it has never been explored.

Kinver Edge

The most recently occupied cave dwellings in Europe are those cut from red sandstone on the borders of north Staffordshire and Worcestershire. At Kinver Edge near Wolverley is the Holy Austin Rock, a large knell which has been excavated to form a number of small chambers, many of them linked by stairways and passages. All are now vacated, but human occupation contained in some of them until the late 1950s - one in particular was a cafe, and the sign *Teas* is still visible there. Another of the strange sandstone outcrops of the area is Nanny's Rock, smaller than Holy Austin Rock but also excavated with a warren of chambers. At the southernmost end of Kinver Edge lies Vale's Rock in which another cave dwelling once existed; not far from this, at the village of Wolverley, is a house built into the rock on which it stands, and at the centre of the village is a cliff which contains the rock-cut habitations of the labourers of a nineteenth-century Iron Master. Many of the cottages built against rock faces in the district had additional rooms excavated in the rock at the back like those on Drury Hill in Nottingham. A small hamlet near Wolverley called Blakeshall had a group of such cottages, and the last to be vacated was at Drakelow, abandoned as late as 1974.

A hermitage complex existed at Arley Kings beside the River Severn, where the monastic ascetics carved many rooms into the red sandstone crags. Today, the whole cliff face is a warren of windows and doorways with the grooves and shaft-holes for door and window shutters still remaining. The twelfth-century priestly poet Layamon, who wrote a notable history of Britain, is reputed to have been an early inhabitant of this hermitage complex, and as late as 1538, on the eve of the suppression of the monasteries, Bishop Latimer wrote that the Arley Kings cave could 'lodge 500 men, as ready for thieves and traitors as true men'.

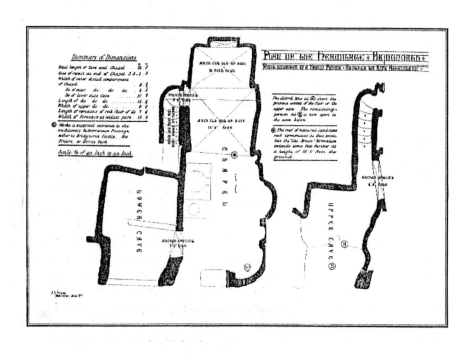

70. Plan of the Hermitage at Bridgnorth, Shropshire,
England. Drawing by A. B. Tinker, 1877. (Nideck)

232

Other religious sites in the district include Southstone Rock at Stanford-on-Teme, where there was a rock-cut chapel dedicated to St John, and the name of Holy Austin Rock itself recalls the legend that St Augustine occupied one of the cells during his missionary expedition of the seventh century.

For the opposition, a large conical mass of sandstone forty feet high called the Devil's Spittleful stands between Kidderminster and Bewdley. This great outcrop, which in legend was a spadeful ('spittleful') dropped by the Devil is honeycombed with ancient rock-cells. Perhaps the site was once associated with the old Pagan religion and the cells may have included a *sacellum* like that at the Externsteine. Many of the cells were occupied until the last century.

Shropshire

The old county of Shropshire had several notable subterranea, some of which survive today. In the east of the county is Tong Castle; the fifth such castle to have occupied the site having been demolished as late as 1954. The earliest castle at Tong was built on the corner of a rocky promontory, and subsequent castles enlarged the site. Beneath them a series of subterranean passages were cut into the red sandstone, linking the cellars with other strategic parts of the building. During the fifteenth to seventeenth centuries the tunnels were part of the defensive system of the castle, but in the eighteenth century the remodelling of the castle by 'Capability' Brown led to their reconstruction as servants' quarters, so that they could live completely underground during the day and not be seen by the owner's aristocratic guests. With little ventilation and by the light of inefficient oil lamps, the life of George Durant's troglodyte servants could not have been pleasant.

At Bridgnorth is The Hermitage, reputed to date from the Saxon period when it was occupied by a brother of King Athelstan. The small cell is carved in soft sandstone, having recesses for a crucifix, lamp, piscina and credence. There are also the remains of several rock-cut arches with rough mouldings rather similar to those found in some of the Nottingham caves. Elsewhere on Hermitage Hill are further rock dwellings and other outcrops in the town are also excavated in like manner. At Downton-on-the- Rock, near Ludlow, a natural cavern was enlarged into an impressive grotto twenty to twenty-five feet in height, containing a spiral column of the type found in the Solomonic/Masonic mysteries, though there is no written or oral record of its function.

Most of the hermitages were abandoned or became secular housing on the suppression of religious orders by Henry VIII. Around the year 1780, a new subterranean religious structure was made in Shropshire at Caynton Hall near Beckbury, where the local landowner made a subterranean temple. Now largely ruined, this consisted of a series of apertures, pillars, alcoves and small chambers carved directly into the sandstone. By 1780, subterranea were no longer anything but quaint conceits for the rich, or hovels for the poor. The Caynton Hall temple is an example of the former.

Yorkshire

The tunnels under York are often mentioned in romantic literature and so it may come as a shock to many that they are part of the more prosaic but nonetheless interesting Roman sewer system. As in so many cities, the redevelopment of parts of the ancient city has uncovered several parts of the network. A typical fragment was discovered on the corner of Church Street and Swinegate in 1972 when workmen struck a large block of stone whilst digging. On removing the block, it was found to be a millstone grit roofing slab of a Roman sewer. Rescue archaeologists were called in, and in December 1972 and January 1973, 145 feet of passages were excavated before foundation work prevented further digging. The 145 foot section running north-west south-east was found to be parallel with the old geomantic Roman street plan, in this

234

case the Via Principalis, but not parallel with any street in the medieval (and modern) layout of York. Only a fragment of the system was explored, but it was found that the passages range from two feet six inches to four feet in height and two feet to three feet seven inches in width. They are lined with blocks of millstone grit, though parts of the sewer's side-passages are lined with limestone ashlars or other types of stone. The date of construction of these passages was not determined, but fragments of debris enabled the archaeologists to estimate that they were last used between the years A.D. 350-400 when the city was in decline.

In about 1918, two residents of Doncaster, H. S. Topham and Dr Renton, noticed a tradesman dumping rubbish down a shaft at the rear of a shop which was built on part of the site of the old Greyfriars Priory. Enquiries revealed that the shop stood over some old cellars, and, some time later, when the shop fell vacant, they decided to investigate. From a range of brick-built cellars, they entered a tunnel six feet six inches high by four feet wide which was arched with stone. About every twenty feet the tunnel had small conical vents entering the roof. The tunnel extended for about forty yards, beyond which it was blocked with earth.

Enquiries revealed that further parts of this tunnel had been found at various times during construction work, and that it must continue right across the town to the river. According to the antiquary Abraham de la Pryme, writing in 1688, the ruins of a religious house at Doncaster contained 'the entrance of a private subterraneous passage which had its direction towards the river and extended a distance of from two to three miles'.

The explanation of this tunnel was that it must have been a Roman sewer, though it must be borne in mind that Doncaster was not a major city like York, which has a somewhat similar system. The vents through the ceiling at

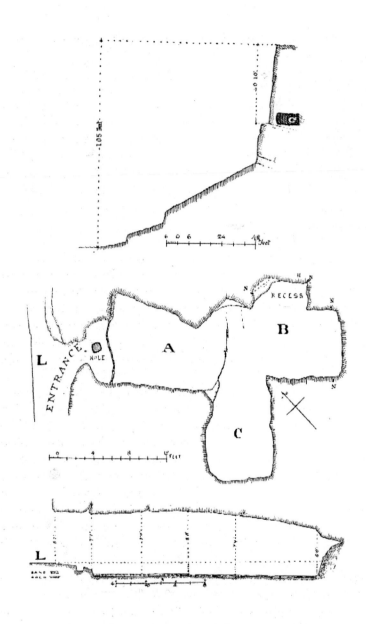

71. Wallace's Cave, Gormerton, Mid Lothian, Scotland.
Drawing by F. R. Coles, 1897. (Nideck)

twenty-foot intervals have still not been convincingly explained.

Rock-cut hermitages existed in Yorkshire at Knaresborough, where several houses in Gracious Street are built onto the front of caves in the time-honoured manner. The caves of Knaresborough were extensive and famous: there is the medieval chapel of Our Lady of the Crag, consecrated in 1409; the cave occupied by the seeress Mother Shipton; the eighteenth-century refuge of Eugene Aram, *The House in the Rock*, a dwelling consisting of several rooms cut out high in a cliff; and the hermitages.

In a garden entered from Back Lane on the outskirts of Pontefract was a most intriguing subterranean hermitage with two chambers and access to underground water by a spiral staircase in a subterranean well beneath a road. The hermitage is notable because its founder, Adam de Laythorpe, is known, for in 1386 he donated some ground belonging to the Friars Preachers to a certain Adam the Hermit for life.

A second chamber existed not far from the first, its entrance being situated about only twenty feet to the west of it. Unlike the first chamber, this was unknown until 1854 when a workman laying a drain penetrated the roof with a pickaxe. The aperture was enlarged, and an entrance made, but public access was not restricted, and by the time the antiquary James Fowler visited it in 1869, vandals had obliterated most of its features. This Pontefract hermitage is most notable for having housed the famous Peter the Hermit who suffered a cruel death under King John for his true and fulfilled prophecy.

Scotland

The most notable series of subterranea in Scotland are found in the valley of the Esk where several complex man-made caves served as habitation and refuge. In construction, some of the caves resemble their counterparts under Nottingham, especially the cave at Gilmerton whose complex structure is accounted for by a tradition that it was built by a smith as his workshop. In the reverend Thomas Whyte's account of Liberton Parish in *Archaeologia Scotica* (1782) we read: 'Here is a famous cave dug out of a rock by one George Paterson, a smith. It was finished in 1724, after five years hard labour .. In this cave are several apartments, several beds, a spacious table with a large punch-bowl, all cut out of the rock in the nicest manner. Here there was a forge, with a well and washing-house.'

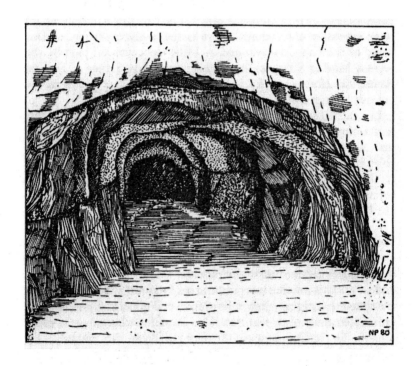

72. Wallace's Cave, Gorston, Scotland. (Nideck)

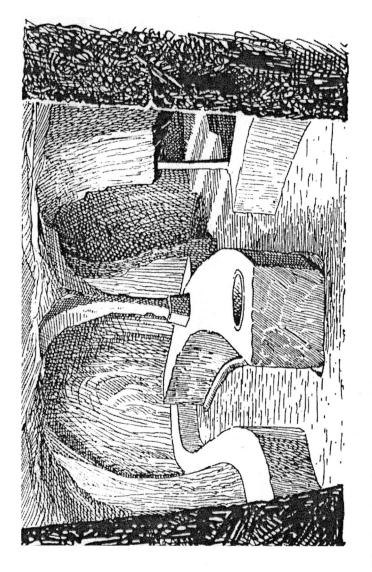

73. The interior of the cave at Gilmerton, Mid Lothian, Scotland. Drawing by F. R. Coles, 1897. (Nideck)

239

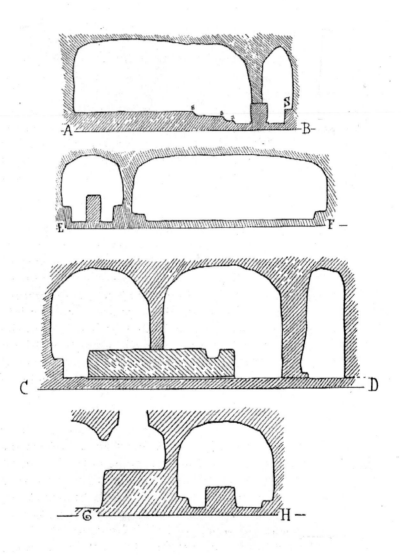

*74. Sections of the cave at Gilmerton, Mid Lothian, Scotland,
Drawings by F. R. Coles, 1897. (Nideck)*

240

The cave was a great tourist attraction in the years after Paterson's death in 1735. Elsewhere in the Esk Valley was an equally famous rock-cut habitation, Wallace's Cave which penetrated the rock for sixty feet. Like the Gorton smithy, it had several architectural features carved from the living rock and was obviously fairly comfortable as far as rock-dwellings go. Nearby, at Hawthornden, the caves were the reputed hiding-place of the Young Pretender in his flight from the English, but that is a common tale for Scottish subterranea. They were in existence in the time of the antiquaries Stukeley and Pennant, who commented on them in their itineraries. Various caves with difficult access were carved in the cliff face, penetrating beneath Hawthornden House as secret escape or access routes.

Elsewhere in Scotland, the earth houses noted above are widespread, but at Dunfermline there exists an important rock-cut hermitage associated with St Margaret, the devout wife of the Scottish King Malcolm Canmore. Now vandalized, this cave was mentioned in Chalmer's *History of Dunfermline,* where 'a person not long since dead (1844) was wont to relate that he knew an aged man who said that he had seen in the cave the remains of a stone table, with something like a crucifix upon it.' The cave still contains the familiar raised ledges or 'seat' found at Nottingham and Gilmerton, and also the customary well.

Another notable artificial subterranean hermitage is St Ringan's Cave, at Billies near Kirkcormack in the Stewartry of Kircudbright. St Ringan is the local name of the hermit St Ninian, the 'Cumbrian Apostle', and his cave has a form very unusual for hermitage use. Carved in the shaly Silurian rock, the cave is entered towards true east, but after about twenty feet it branches towards true north. This branch proceeds for another thirty feet, after which it deviates to the north-west. In structure it is similar to the tunnel which links two cottages at Fowlmere in Cambridgeshire, though it ends in a seat-like recess 115 feet from the entrance. It does not resemble the conventional hermitage, and may have served some oracular function with the early Celtic saint in attendance.

Postscript

In this final section I have only been able to touch upon a few of the most notable of thousands of subterranea which lurk beneath the ground of this country. Most of the features of such tunnels and networks are similar, however, I have dealt with all of the characteristic types encountered in these isles and elsewhere. There are many reports and accounts of specific tunnel and cave systems, and in the bibliography I list the major sources and books which might prove the most useful to those who wish to continue the study of a most worthwhile field of investigation. Although the well-known and easily accessible subterranea are fascinating, the greatest challenge is in those yet to be found. As I was writing the first edition, a tunnel over 100 feet long has opened up beneath a primary school in Great Cornard in Suffolk and the residents of a nearby housing estate believe that a chalk mine like that at Bury St Edmunds may exist beneath their properties. Since then, a double-decker bus has fallen through a Norwich street, and many similar instances of subsidence have been attributed to subterranea. The subterranean kingdom still makes its presence known in the most unexpected ways.

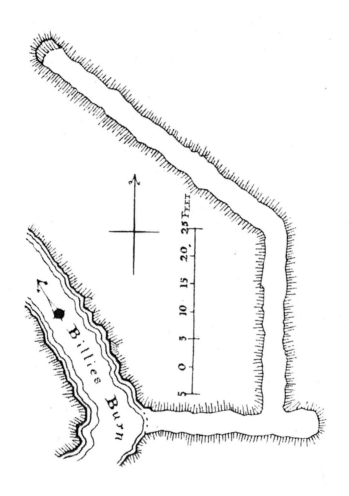

76. *The kind of caves used by the Celtic saints is typified by St. Ringan's Cave at Billie's Burn, Kirkcormack. In the Stewartry of Kirkcudbright, Scotland. Plan by F. R. Coles, 1897. (Nideck)*

Bibliography

Agricola, Georgius. *De Re Metallica* (1556).
Anderson, J. *Scotland in Pagan Times*(1883).
Apollodorus. *The Library*.
Asser. *The Life Of King Alfred*.
Bayley, Harold. *Archaic England* (London, 1919).
Bedford, Bruce; Underground Britain. (London, 1985).
Bond, Frederick Bligh. *Glastonbury Abbey* (Glastonbury, 1920).
Borlase, William. *The Antiquities of Cornwall* (1754).
Breasted, James. *A History of Egypt* (London, 1909).
Broens, M. Ces Souterrains: *Refuges pour les vivants, or pour les esprits?*(Paris, 1976).
Camden, W. *Britannia* (London, 1610).
Carroll, Lewis. *Alice's Adventures in Wonderland* (London, 1865).
Clarke, Evelyn. *Cornish Fogous*(London, 1961).
Clay, Rotha Mary. *The Hermits and Anchorites of England* (London, 1914).
Crawford, Harriet (ed.): *Subterranean Britain, aspects of underground archaeology*. (London 1979).
Dall, W. H. *On the Remains of Later Prehistoric Man Obtained Fromthe Caves of the Aleutian Islands* (Washington City, 1878).
Davies, O.: *Roman Mines of Europe*. (Oxford, 1935).
Deering,Charles. *The History of Nottinghamshire* Nottingham,1751).
Devereux, P. and Thomson, I. *The Ley Hunter's Companion* (London, 1979).
Dickens, Charles. *The Pickwick Papers*.
Emerson, William G. *The Smoky God*.
Fea, J. Allen. *Rooms of Mystery and Romance* (London, 1923).
Fells, Richard: *A Visitor's Guide to Underground Britain*. (London, 1989).
Hall, Captain. *Life with the Esquimaux* (London, 1864).
Hencken, H. O'N. *The Archaeology of Cornwall and Scilly* (London, 1932).
Herodotus. *The Histories*.
Lambarde, William.*The Perambulation of Kent*(London, 1570).
Le Poer Trench, Brinsley. *The Secret of the Ages: UFOs From Inside the Earth* (London, 1974).
Levi, Eliphas. *The History of Magic* (London, 1913).

244

Lloyd, John Uri. *Etidorhpa, or the End of the Earth* (1895).
Lytton, Lord Bulwer. *The Coming Race* (London, 1871).
MacCulloch, A. *The Statistical Account* (Wigtown, 1841).
MacTaggart, John. *The Scottish Gallovidian Encyclopaedia* (London, 1824).
Nance, R. M. *Cornish-English Dictionary* (1955).
Nilsson, Sven. *The Primitive Inhabitants of Scandinavia* (London, 1868).
Northcote, J. Spencer. *The Roman Catacombs* (London, 1856).
Ossendowski, Ferdinand. *Beasts, Men and Gods* (London, 1923).
Pennick, Ann. *Deneholes and Subterranea* (Bar Hill, 1975).
Pennick, Nigel. *The Mysteries of King's College Chapel* (Thorsons,1978).
- - . *The Ancient Science of Geomancy* (London, 1979).
Plot, Robert. *The Natural History of Oxfordshire* (1705).
Pollo, M. Vitruvius. *The Ten Books on Architecture.*
Reed, William. *The Phantom of the Poles* (London, 1906).
Roberts, Anthony (editor). *Glastonbury - Ancient Avalon, New Jerusalem* (London, 1978).
Roberts, Anthony, and Gilbertson, Geoff.*The Dark Gods* (London,1980).
Roerich, Nicholas. *Shambhala* (London, 1930).
Scott, Sir Walter. *Marmion.*
Screeton, Paul. *Quicksilver Heritage* (Thorsons, 1974).
Spence, Lewis. *The Mysteries of Britain* (Aquarian Press, 1979).
Squiers, Granville. *Secret Hiding Places*(London, 1933). Stockdale, W. *The Survey of the Lands of the Percies* (1586). Stowe, John. *The Survey of London* (1581).
Strassburg, Gottfried von. *Tristan* (c. 1210).
Teudt, Wilhelm. *Germanische Heiligtumer* (Jena, 1929).
Tudor, J. R. *The Orkneys and Shetland* (London, 1883).
Urwin, J. Hope. *Secret Hiding Places and Underground Passages* (London, 1936).
Verne, Jules. *A Journey to the Centre of the Earth.*
Virgil. *The Aenid.*
Watkins, Alfred. *The Old Straight Track* (London, 1925).
Wells, H. G. *The Time Machine* (London, 1899).
Wilkins, Harold T. *The Mysteries of Ancient South America* (London, 1945).
Williams, F.R. *Anstey - A Hertfordshire Parish* (Cambridge, 1929)
Williams, R. *Lexicon Cornu - Britannicum* (Landovery, 1865)
Windle, Sir Bertram, *Life in Early Britain.* (London, 1895).
Wood, J Maxwell. *Witchcraft and Superstitious Record in the South-Western District of Scotland* (1911).
Woodbridge, Kenneth: *Landscape and Antiquity.* (Oxford, 1970).

Anonymous Ancient Sources
The Collquy of Archbishop Aelfric.
The Chronicles of Hyde Abbey.
The Legend of Sawney Beane (Broadsheet c. 1700)
The Magical Oracles of Zoroaster.
The Orkneying Saga (12th century).
The Rule for Hermits.
Tristramssaga (1226).
Sir Tristram (13th century).

Journals Consulted
Archaeology
The Antiquaries' Journal
The Archaeological Journal.
Ancient Mysteries.
British Archaeological Association Journal.
Bulletin of Subterranea Britannica.
The Cambrian Register.
Cambridge News.
Coal Age.
Concrete and Constructional Engineering.
The East Anglian Daily Times.
The Engineer.
The Journal of Geomancy.
The Journal of The Royal Society of Antiquaries, Ireland.
Kent Trust Bulletin.
Lantern (Lowestoft).
The Ley Hunter.
Notes and Queries.
The Post Office Courier.
Proceedings of the Geological Association.
The Reliquary.
The Scotsman.
Smithsonian Contributions to Knowledge.

Glossary

Adit. Entrance to a mine by a more or less horizontal passage.

Bell Pit. An early method of mining, using a vertical shaft with the bottom 'belled out' in the seam to be mined.

Canch Working. Bottom or top canch, a form of tunnel construction where the rock is excavated from the bottom or top first, leaving a bench (bottom canch) or an overhang (top canch).

Catacomb. Underground tunnel used for the burial of the dead.

Chalk Well. Method of obtaining agricultural chalk using a vertical shaft leading to short galleries, usually collapsed deliberately when exhausted.

Creep. Narrow and low side tunnel, perhaps used for ventilation purposes or escape, found in earth houses and fogous.

Crypt. Underground or semi-underground shrine room beneath the high altar of a church or cathedral.

Cut-and-cover. Tunnelling method involving digging a trench then roofing it over.

Denehole. A vertical-shafted structure cut through overlying sands into chalk, in which vaulted rooms, but not tunnels, were excavated.

Earth House. Scottish term for a man-made underground structure primarily used for habitation. Sometimes known as Picts' Houses.

Fogou. Cornish underground structure resembling Scottish earth houses but perhaps with ritual use.

Geomancy. The placing of sacred buildings in a specific relationship with others with regard to geometry, orientation and astrological conditions.

Grotto. A small, usually artificial cave, often lined with seashells or other decoration, originally derived from shrines to St James the Greater.

Hermitage. Habitation of a religious recluse, usually incorporating a chapel or oratory.

Hollow Earth Theory. Theory that the planet Earth has holes at the poles which lead into an unexpected inner world.

Hypogeum. Subterranean building, generally for religious use.

Ley (ley-line). An alignment of ancient sites believed to be deliberately laid out in antiquity for geomantic purposes.

Lime Blasting. Mining technique using the explosive properties of quicklime.

Lime House. Excavation in industrial waste for habitation at Buxton, Derbyshire.

Luminare. Subterranean tomb or chapel illuminated by a light tube from the surface.

Metro. Largely underground urban railway system, named after the world's first, London Metropolitan Railway (1863).

Omphalos. Literally, the navel of the world, a central point around which all other places are arranged.

Ossorium. Subterranean repository for the bones of the dead.

Sacellum. A small Pagan chapel.

Shaft. A vertical opening in the ground.

Sough. Tunnel driven specifically to drain a mine. *Souterrain.* French term for man-made underground structure used for habitation, storage or ritual, also used to describe Irish examples.

Stannary. The independent parliament of the tin miners of Cornwall .

Steining (steyning or *steening).* Lining of a well, either of brick, stone or wood.

Tube Tunnel. A tunnel bored through rock or clay using a lining of cast iron or concrete (post-1869).

Uaimh (pronounced oo-av). An Irish earth house (Scottish Gaelic equivalent *uamh,* pronounced weem).

FREE DETAILED CATALOGUE

Capall Bann is owned and run by people actively involved in many of the areas in which we publish. A detailed illustrated catalogue is available on request, SAE or International Postal Coupon appreciated. **Titles can be ordered direct from Capall Bann, post free in the UK** (cheque or PO with order) or from good bookshops and specialist outlets.

Do contact us for details on the latest releases at: **Capall Bann Publishing, Freshfields, Chieveley, Berks, RG20 8TF.** Titles include:

A Breath Behind Time, Terri Hector
Angels and Goddesses - Celtic Christianity & Paganism, M. Howard
Arthur - The Legend Unveiled, C Johnson & E Lung
Astrology The Inner Eye - A Guide in Everyday Language, E Smith
Auguries and Omens - The Magical Lore of Birds, Yvonne Aburrow
Asyniur - Womens Mysteries in the Northern Tradition, S McGrath
Beginnings - Geomancy, Builder's Rites & Electional Astrology in the
      European Tradition, Nigel Pennick
Between Earth and Sky, Julia Day
Book of the Veil , Peter Paddon
Caer Sidhe - Celtic Astrology and Astronomy, Vol 1, Michael Bayley
Caer Sidhe - Celtic Astrology and Astronomy, Vol 2 M Bayley
Call of the Horned Piper, Nigel Jackson
Cat's Company, Ann Walker
Celtic Faery Shamanism, Catrin James
Celtic Faery Shamanism - The Wisdom of the Otherworld, Catrin James
Celtic Lore & Druidic Ritual, Rhiannon Ryall
Celtic Sacrifice - Pre Christian Ritual & Religion, Marion Pearce
Celtic Saints and the Glastonbury Zodiac, Mary Caine
Circle and the Square, Jack Gale
Compleat Vampyre - The Vampyre Shaman, Nigel Jackson
Creating Form From the Mist - The Wisdom of Women in Celtic Myth and
      Culture, Lynne Sinclair-Wood
Crystal Clear - A Guide to Quartz Crystal, Jennifer Dent
Crystal Doorways, Simon & Sue Lilly
Crossing the Borderlines - Guising, Masking & Ritual Animal Disguise in the
      European Tradition, Nigel Pennick
Dragons of the West, Nigel Pennick
Earth Dance - A Year of Pagan Rituals, Jan Brodie
Earth Harmony - Places of Power, Holiness & Healing, Nigel Pennick
Earth Magic, Margaret McArthur

Eildon Tree (The) Romany Language & Lore, Michael Hoadley
Enchanted Forest - The Magical Lore of Trees, Yvonne Aburrow
Eternal Priestess, Sage Weston
Eternally Yours Faithfully, Roy Radford & Evelyn Gregory
Everything You Always Wanted To Know About Your Body, But So Far
    Nobody's Been Able To Tell You, Chris Thomas & D Baker
Face of the Deep - Healing Body & Soul, Penny Allen
Fairies in the Irish Tradition, Molly Gowen
Familiars - Animal Powers of Britain, Anna Franklin
Fool's First Steps, (The) Chris Thomas
Forest Paths - Tree Divination, Brian Harrison, Ill. S. Rouse
From Past to Future Life, Dr Roger Webber
Gardening For Wildlife Ron Wilson
God Year, The, Nigel Pennick & Helen Field
Goddess on the Cross, Dr George Young
Goddess Year, The, Nigel Pennick & Helen Field
Goddesses, Guardians & Groves, Jack Gale
Handbook For Pagan Healers, Liz Joan
Handbook of Fairies, Ronan Coghlan
Healing Book, The, Chris Thomas and Diane Baker
Healing Homes, Jennifer Dent
Healing Journeys, Paul Williamson
Healing Stones, Sue Philips
Herb Craft - Shamanic & Ritual Use of Herbs, Lavender & Franklin
Hidden Heritage - Exploring Ancient Essex, Terry Johnson
Hub of the Wheel, Skytoucher
In Search of Herne the Hunter, Eric Fitch
Inner Celtia, Alan Richardson & David Annwn
Inner Mysteries of the Goths, Nigel Pennick
Inner Space Workbook - Develop Thru Tarot, C Summers & J Vayne
Intuitive Journey, Ann Walker Isis - African Queen, Akkadia Ford
Journey Home, The, Chris Thomas
Kecks, Keddles & Kesh - Celtic Lang & The Cog Almanac, Bayley
Language of the Psycards, Berenice
Legend of Robin Hood, The, Richard Rutherford-Moore
Lid Off the Cauldron, Patricia Crowther
Light From the Shadows - Modern Traditional Witchcraft, Gwyn
Living Tarot, Ann Walker
Lore of the Sacred Horse, Marion Davies
Lost Lands & Sunken Cities (2nd ed.), Nigel Pennick
Magic of Herbs - A Complete Home Herbal, Rhiannon Ryall
Magical Guardians - Exploring the Spirit and Nature of Trees, Philip Heselton
Magical History of the Horse, Janet Farrar & Virginia Russell
Magical Lore of Animals, Yvonne Aburrow
Magical Lore of Cats, Marion Davies
Magical Lore of Herbs, Marion Davies

Magick Without Peers, Ariadne Rainbird & David Rankine
Masks of Misrule - Horned God & His Cult in Europe, Nigel Jackson
Medicine For The Coming Age, Lisa Sand MD
Medium Rare - Reminiscences of a Clairvoyant, Muriel Renard
Menopausal Woman on the Run, Jaki da Costa
Mind Massage - 60 Creative Visualisations, Marlene Maundrill
Mirrors of Magic - Evoking the Spirit of the Dewponds, P Heselton
Moon Mysteries, Jan Brodie
Mysteries of the Runes, Michael Howard
Mystic Life of Animals, Ann Walker
New Celtic Oracle The, Nigel Pennick & Nigel Jackson
Oracle of Geomancy, Nigel Pennick
Pagan Feasts - Seasonal Food for the 8 Festivals, Franklin & Phillips
Patchwork of Magic - Living in a Pagan World, Julia Day
Pathworking - A Practical Book of Guided Meditations, Pete Jennings
Personal Power, Anna Franklin
Pickingill Papers - The Origins of Gardnerian Wicca, Bill Liddell
Pillars of Tubal Cain, Nigel Jackson
Places of Pilgrimage and Healing, Adrian Cooper
Practical Divining, Richard Foord
Practical Meditation, Steve Hounsome
Practical Spirituality, Steve Hounsome
Psychic Self Defence - Real Solutions, Jan Brodie
Real Fairies, David Tame
Reality - How It Works & Why It Mostly Doesn't, Rik Dent
Romany Tapestry, Michael Houghton
Runic Astrology, Nigel Pennick
Sacred Animals, Gordon MacLellan
Sacred Celtic Animals, Marion Davies, Ill. Simon Rouse
Sacred Dorset - On the Path of the Dragon, Peter Knight
Sacred Grove - The Mysteries of the Forest, Yvonne Aburrow
Sacred Geometry, Nigel Pennick
Sacred Nature, Ancient Wisdom & Modern Meanings, A Cooper
Sacred Ring - Pagan Origins of British Folk Festivals, M. Howard
Season of Sorcery - On Becoming a Wisewoman, Poppy Palin
Seasonal Magic - Diary of a Village Witch, Paddy Slade
Secret Places of the Goddess, Philip Heselton
Secret Signs & Sigils, Nigel Pennick
Self Enlightenment, Mayan O'Brien
Spirits of the Air, Jaq D Hawkins
Spirits of the Earth, Jaq D Hawkins
Spirits of the Earth, Jaq D Hawkins
Stony Gaze, Investigating Celtic Heads John Billingsley
Stumbling Through the Undergrowth , Mark Kirwan-Heyhoe
Subterranean Kingdom, The, revised 2nd ed, Nigel Pennick
Symbols of Ancient Gods, Rhiannon Ryall

FREE detailed catalogue and FREE 'Inspiration' magazine

Contact: Capall Bann Publishing, Freshfields, Chieveley, Berks, RG20 8TF